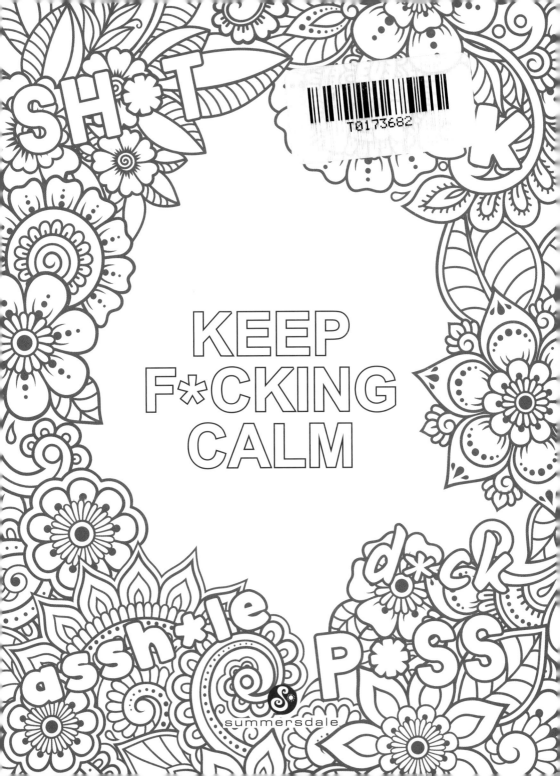

SH*T

K

KEEP
F*CKING
CALM

d*ck

assh*le

P*SS

summersdale

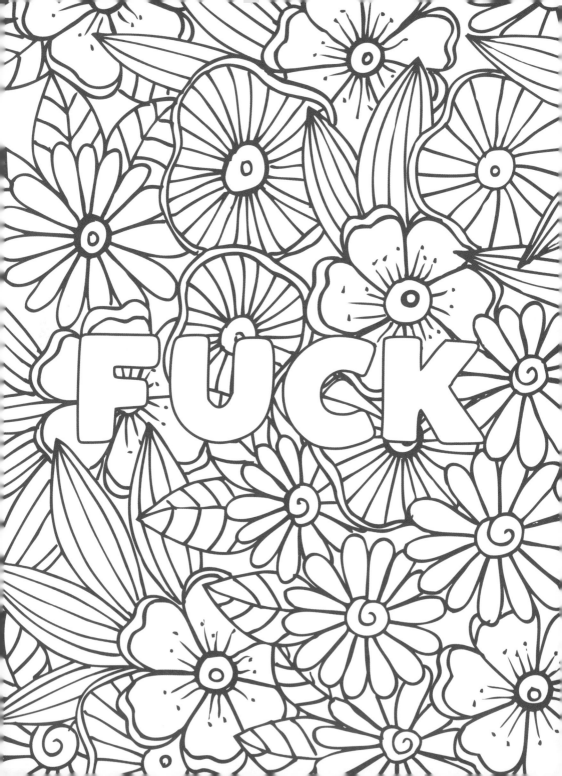

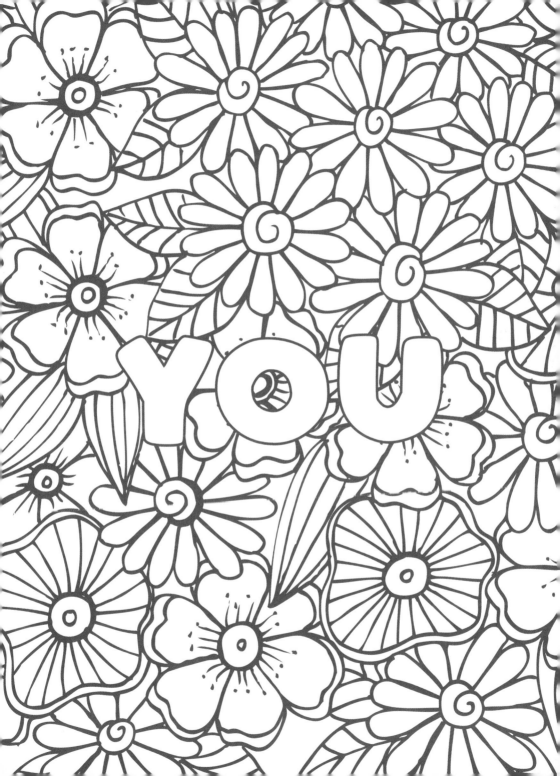

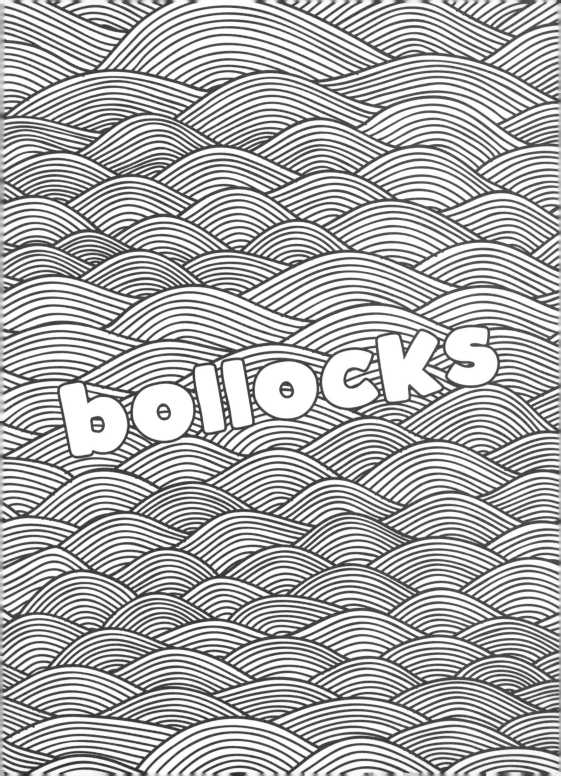

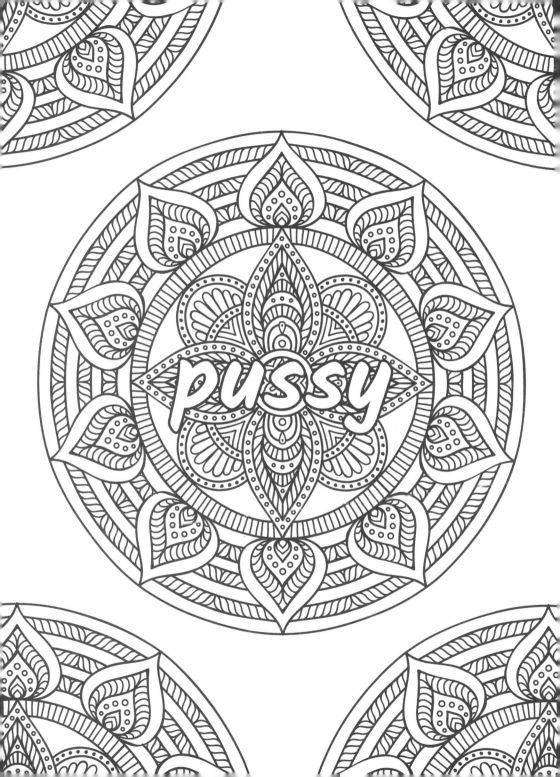

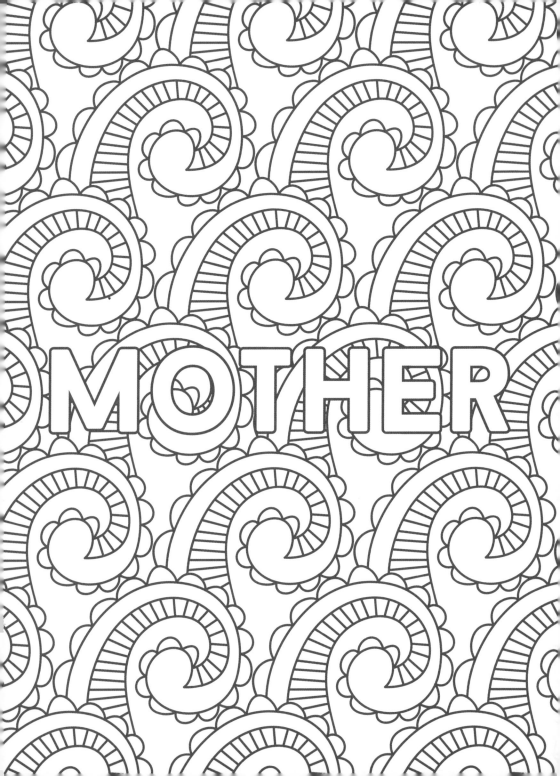

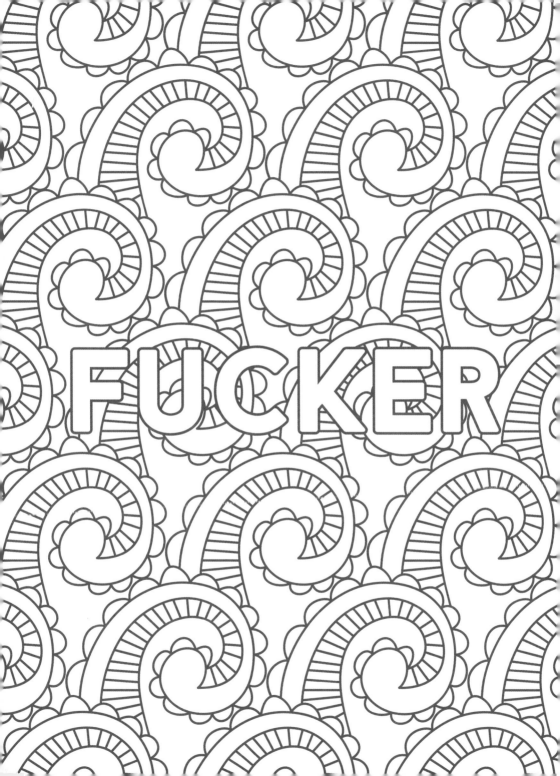

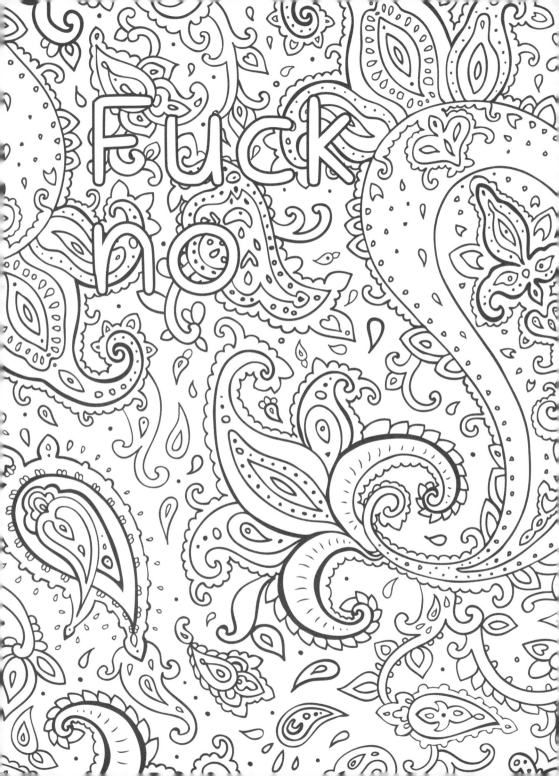

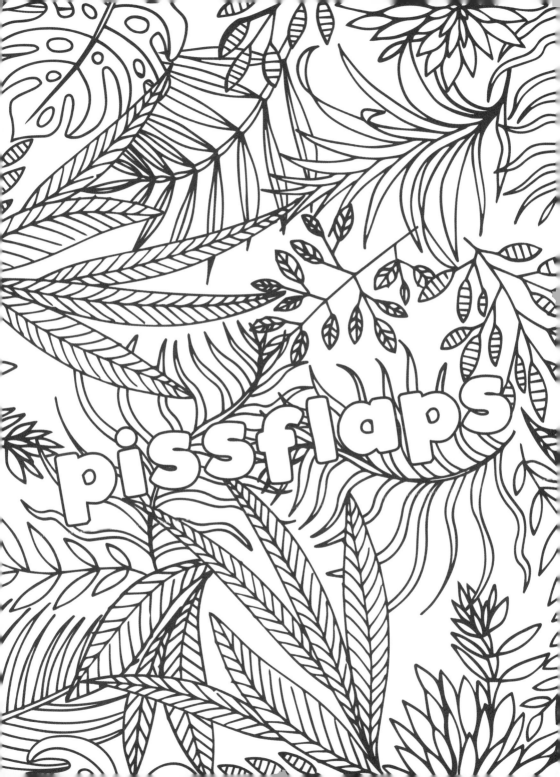

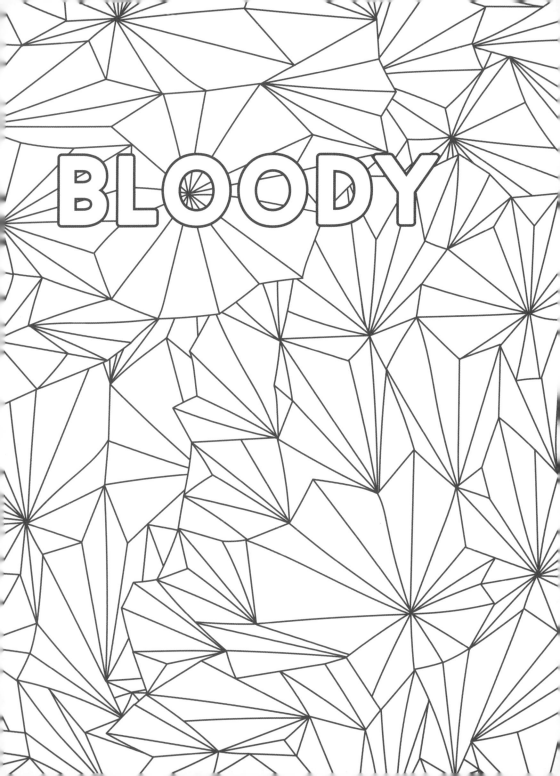

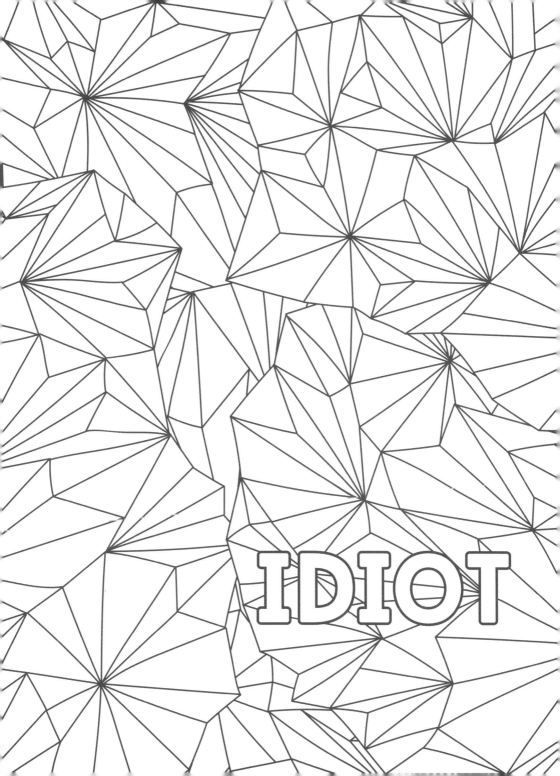

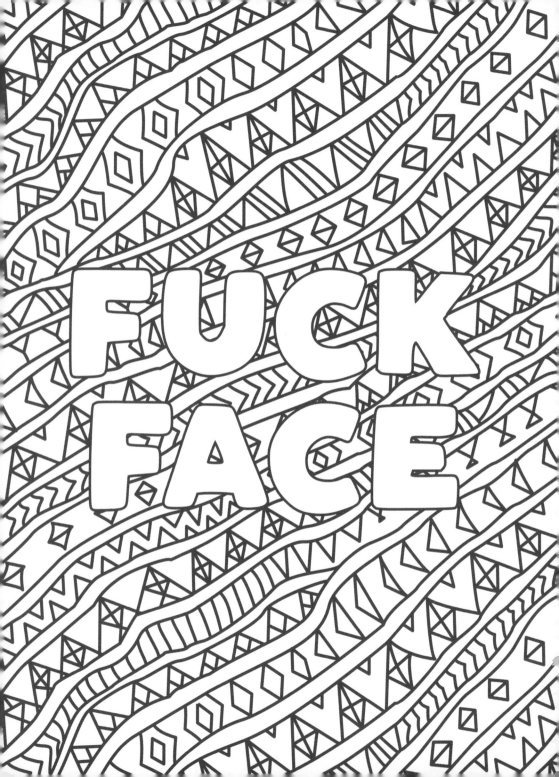

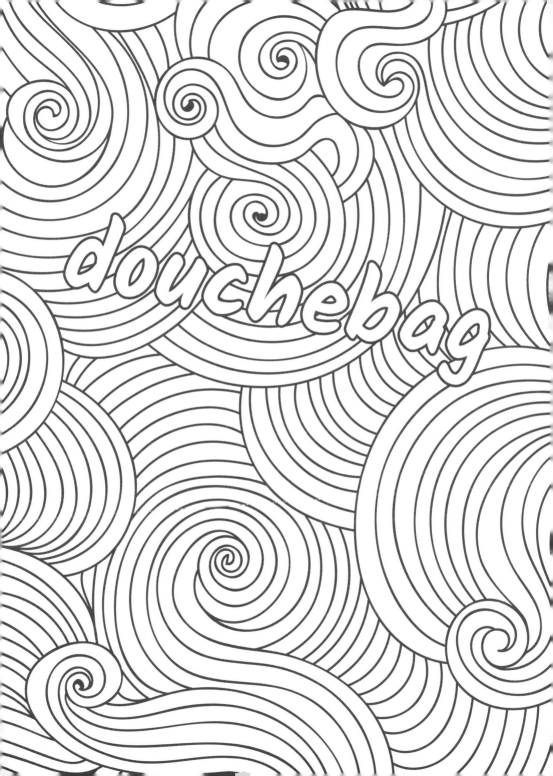

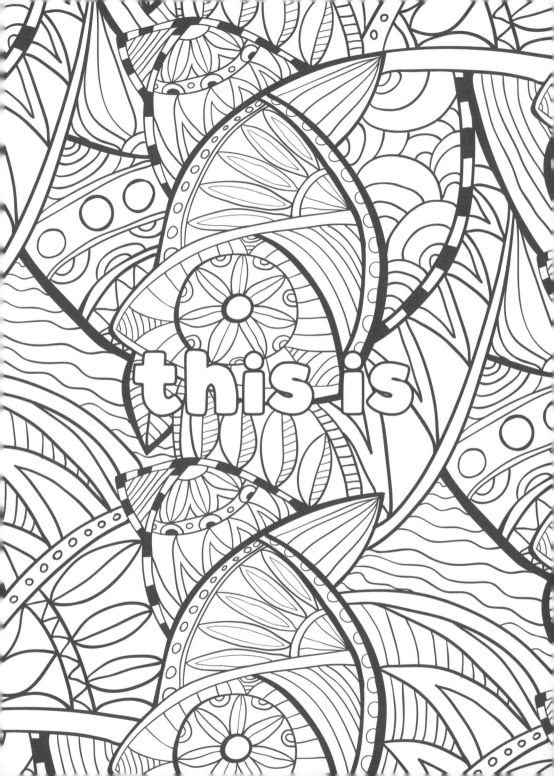

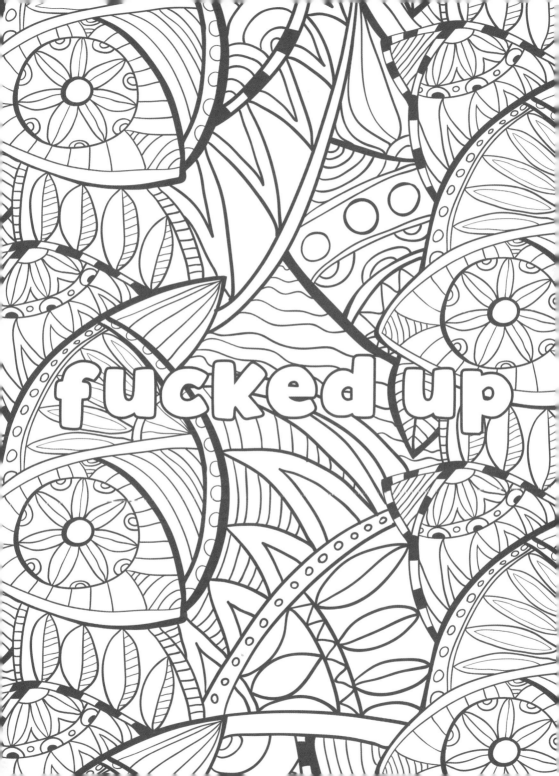

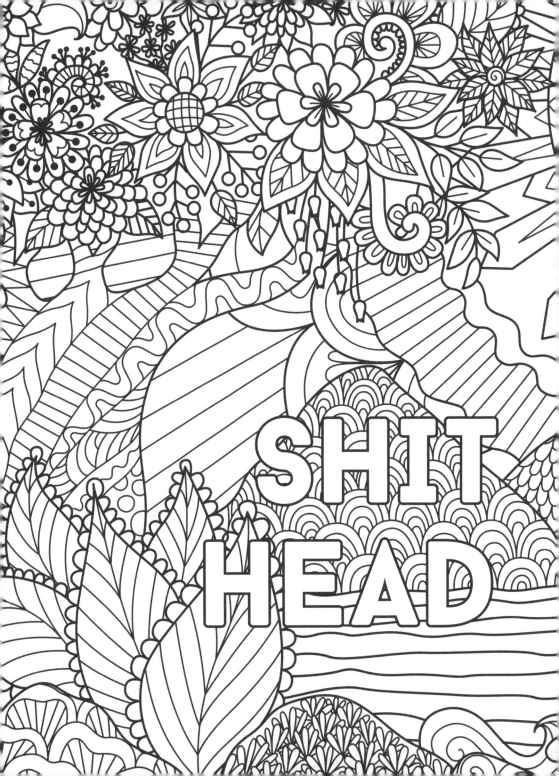

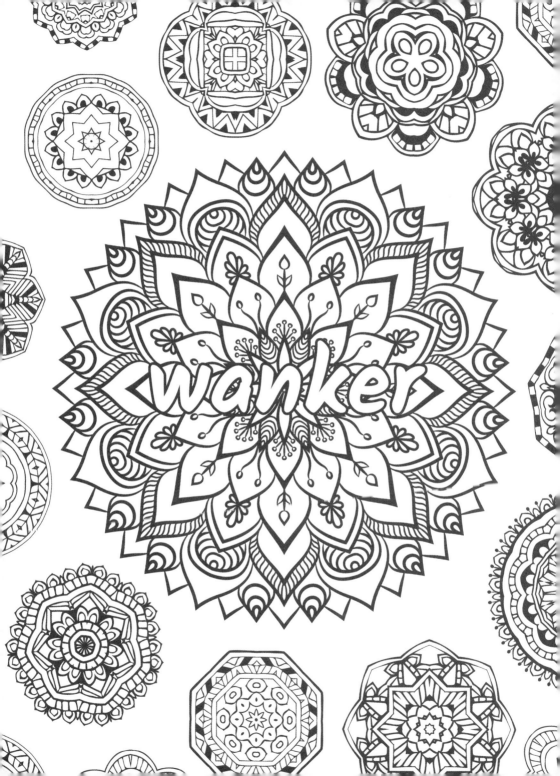

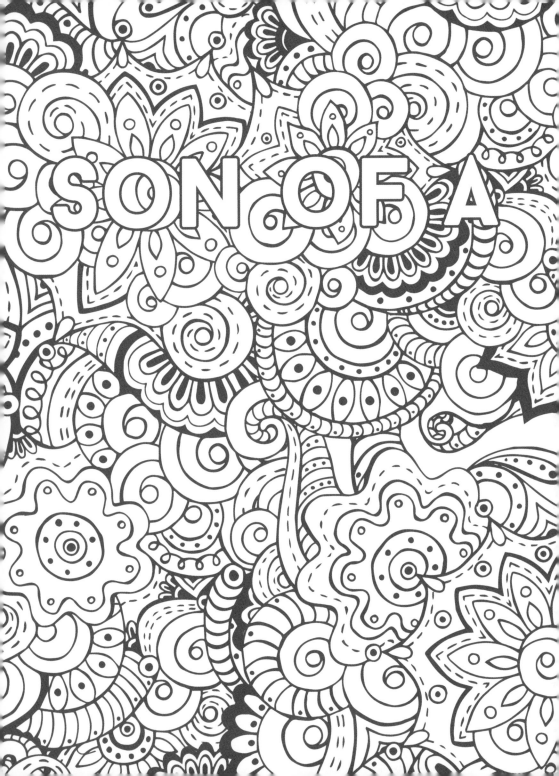

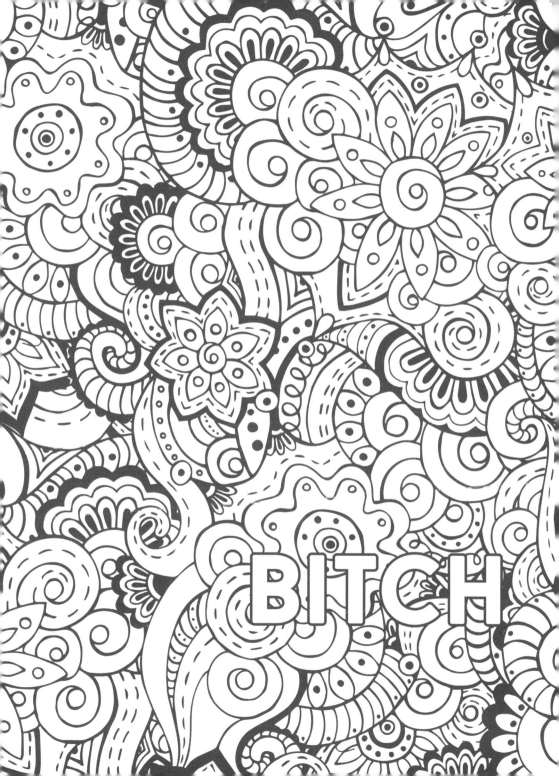

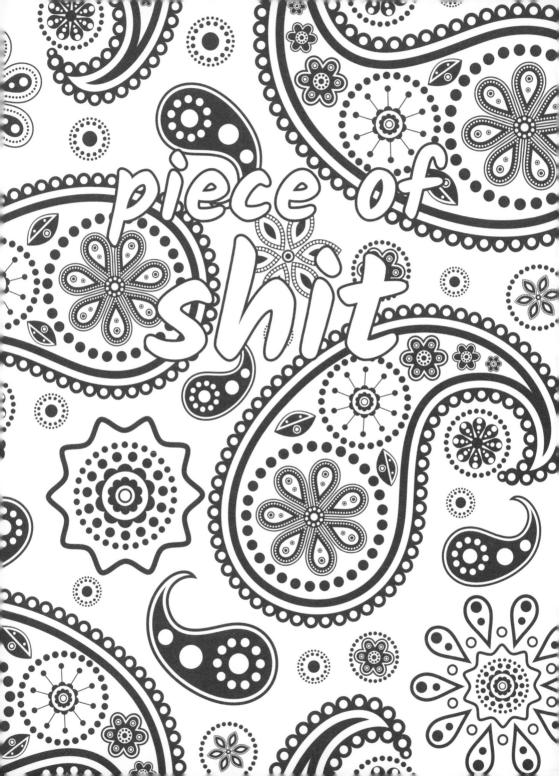

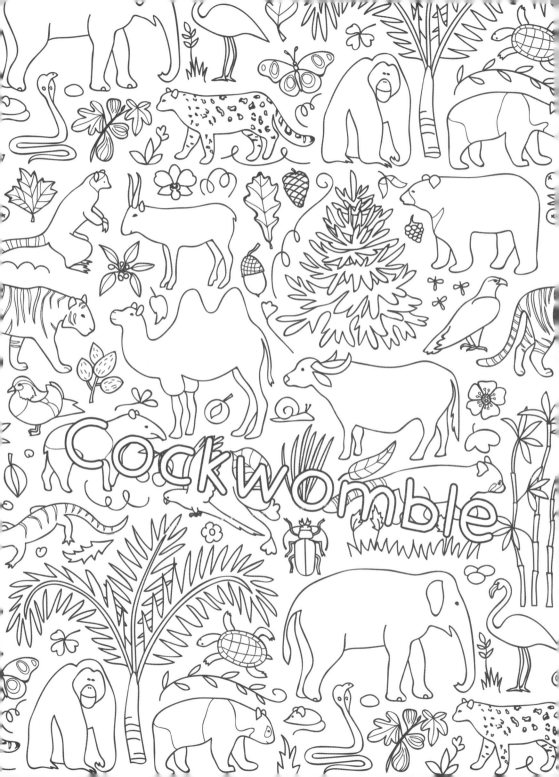

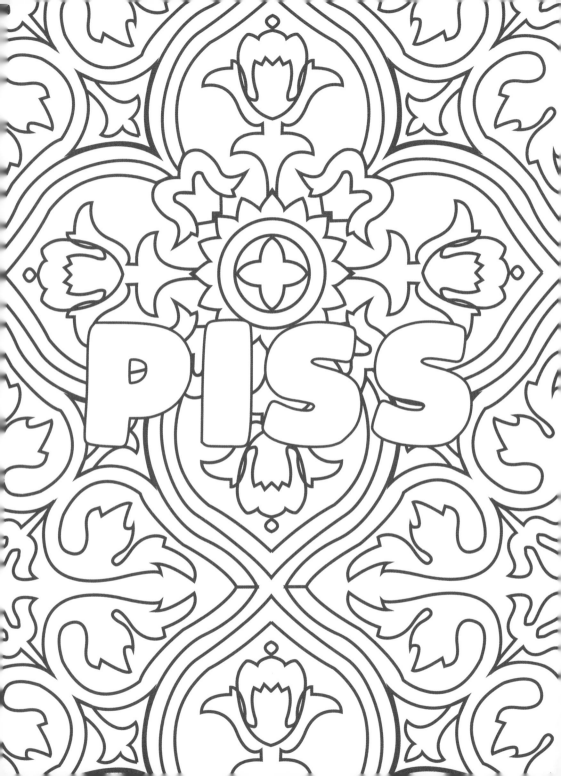

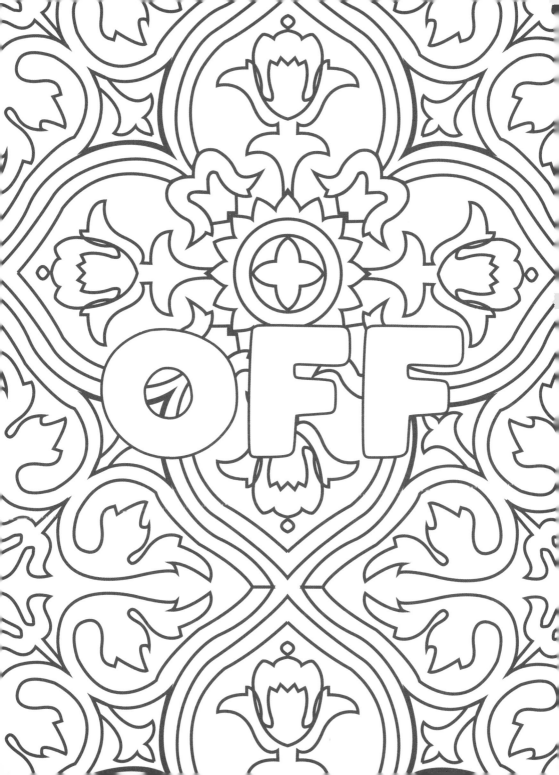

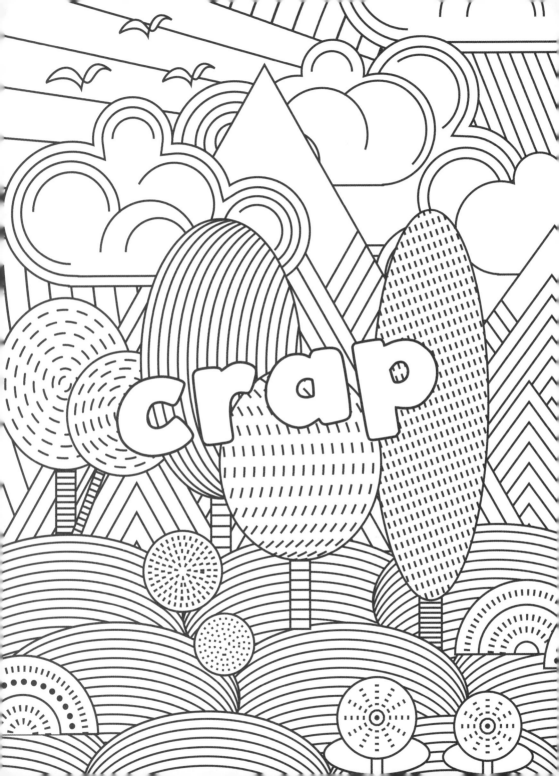

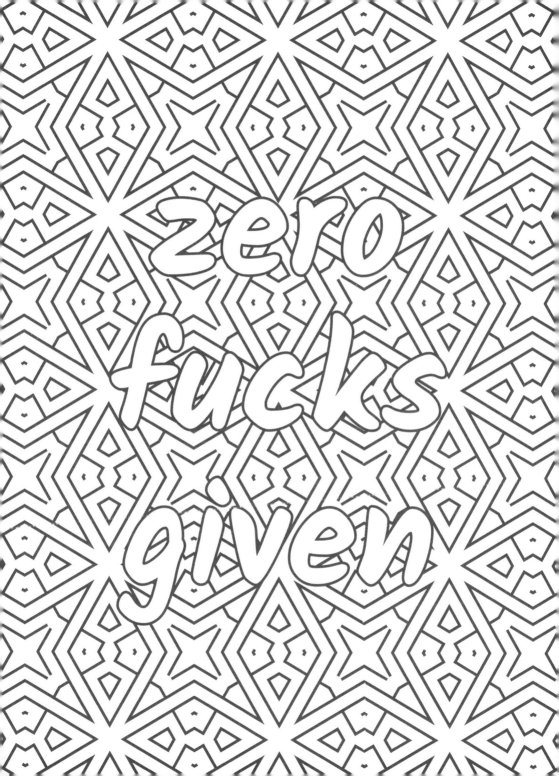

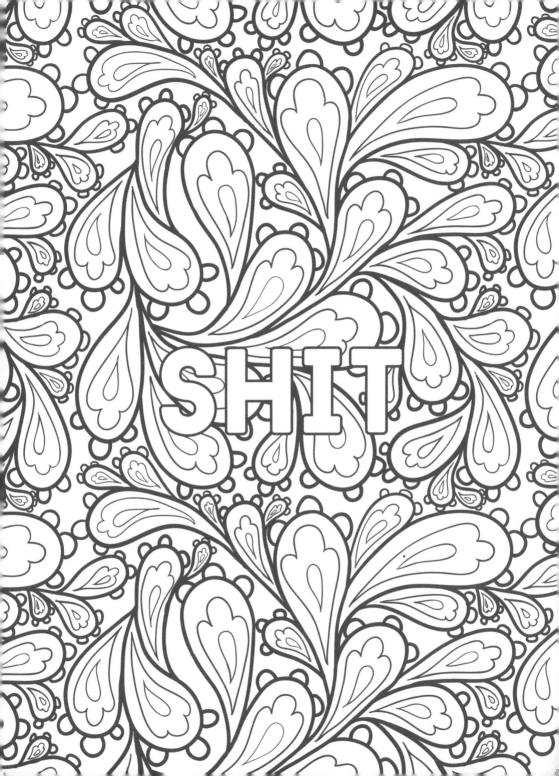

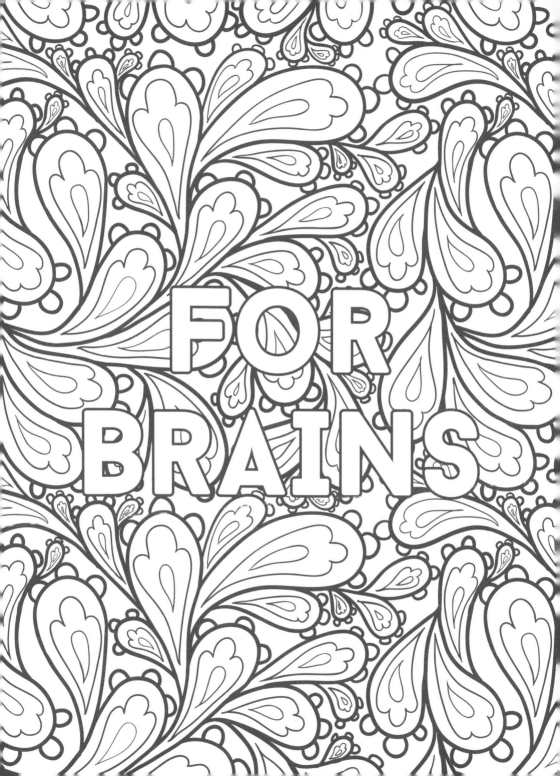

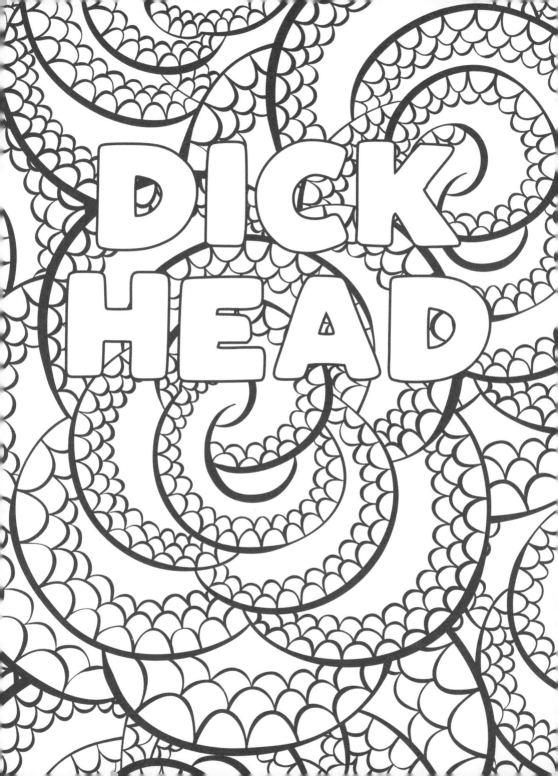

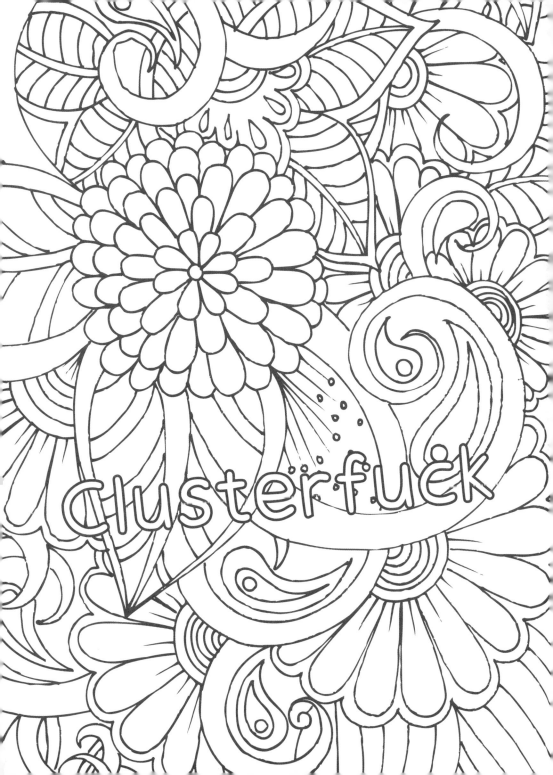

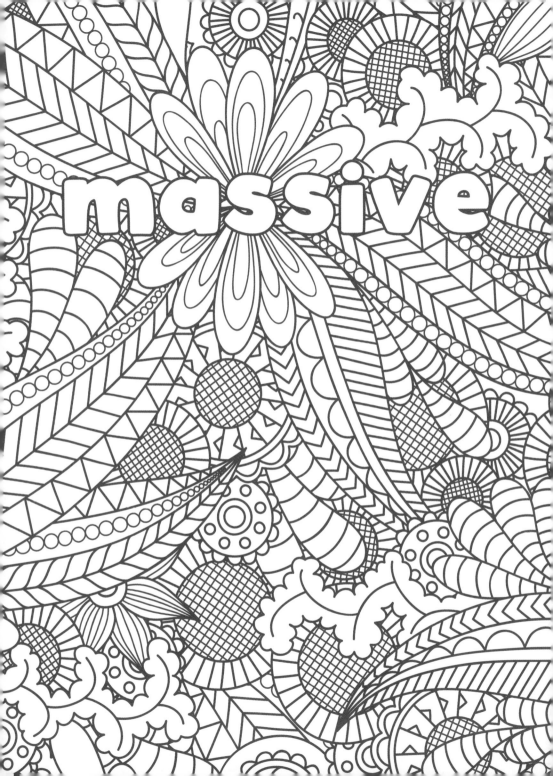

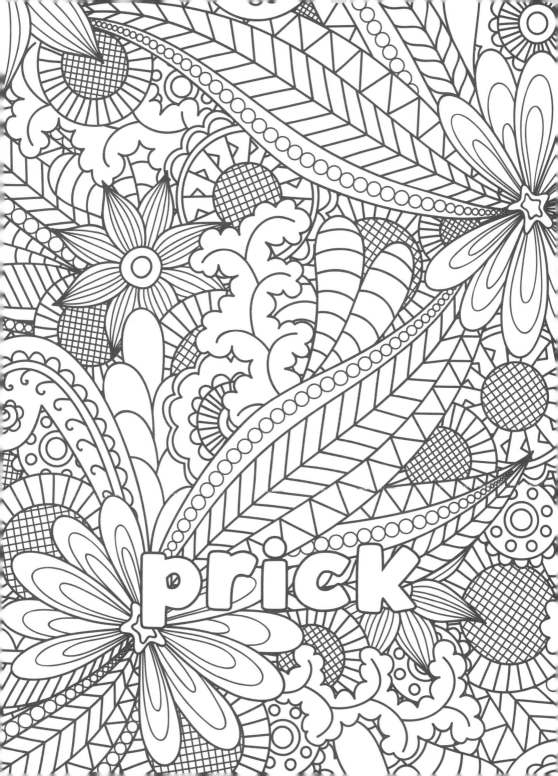

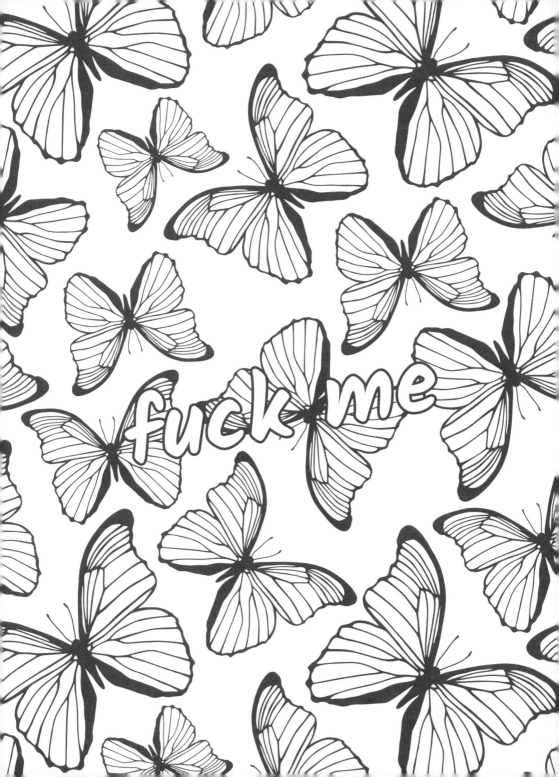

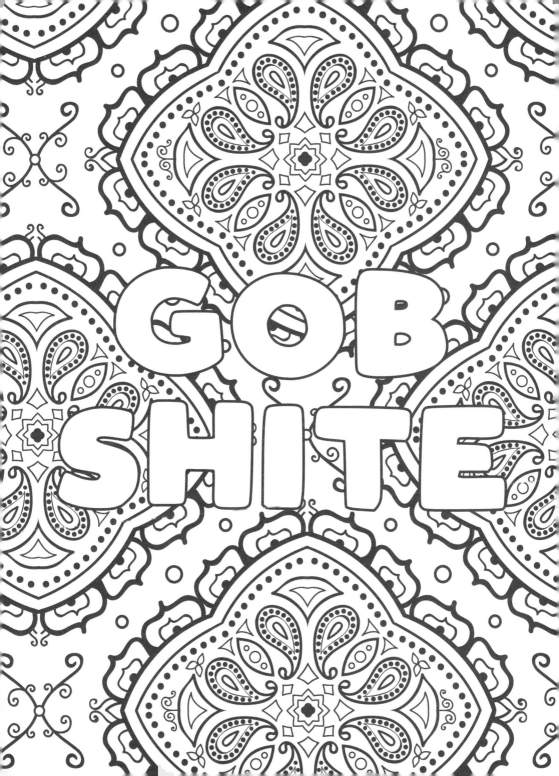

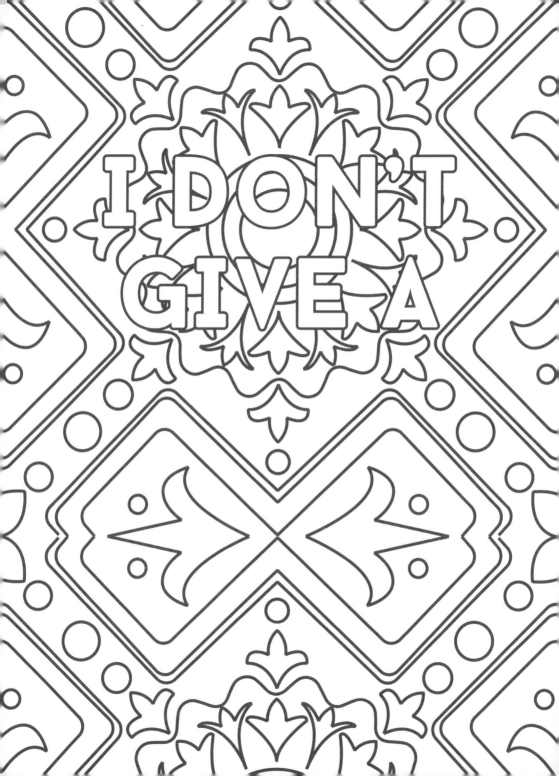

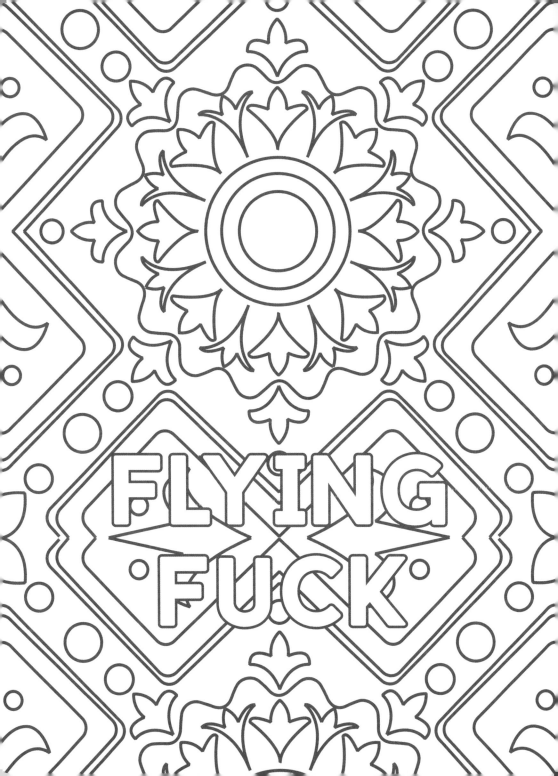

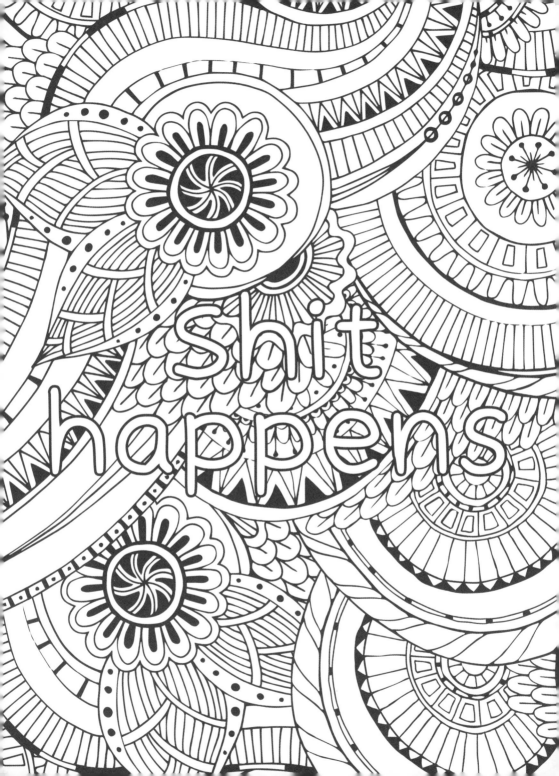

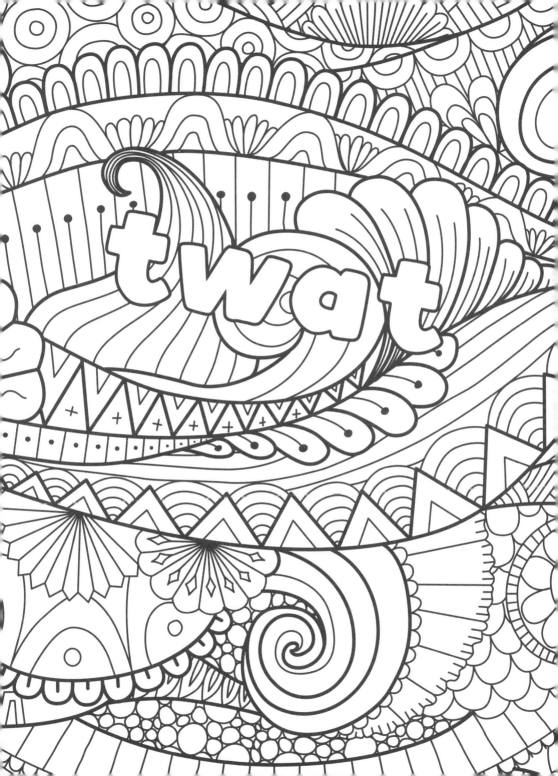

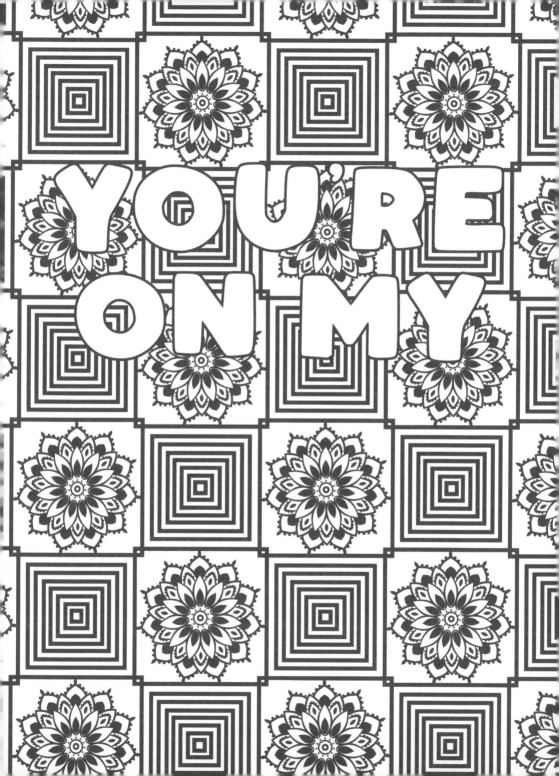

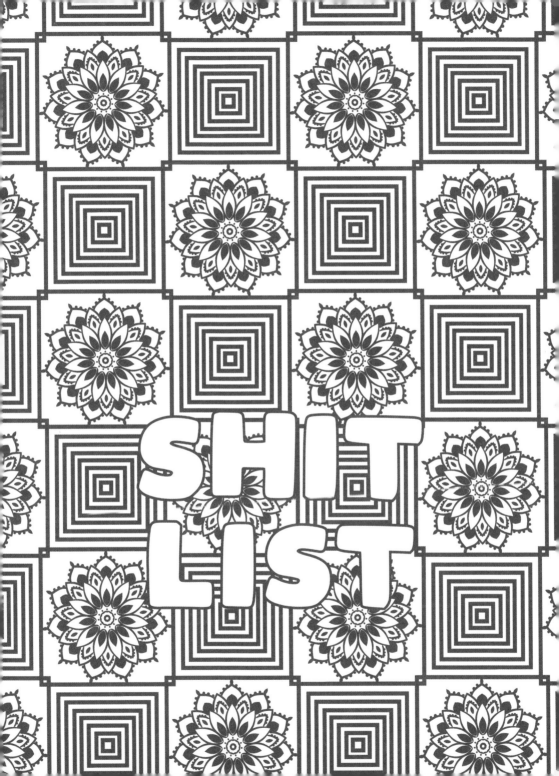

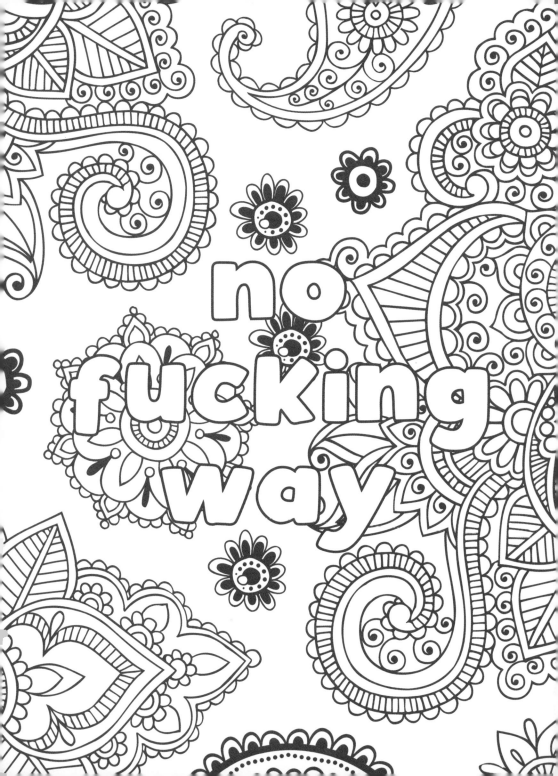

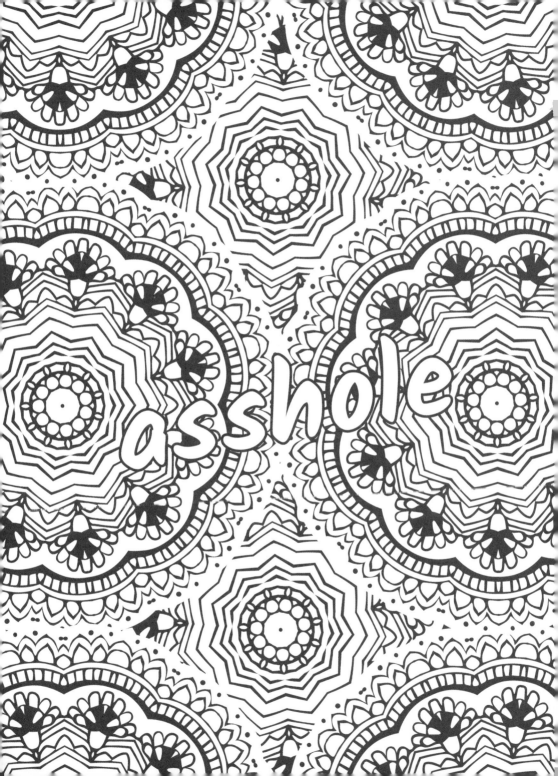

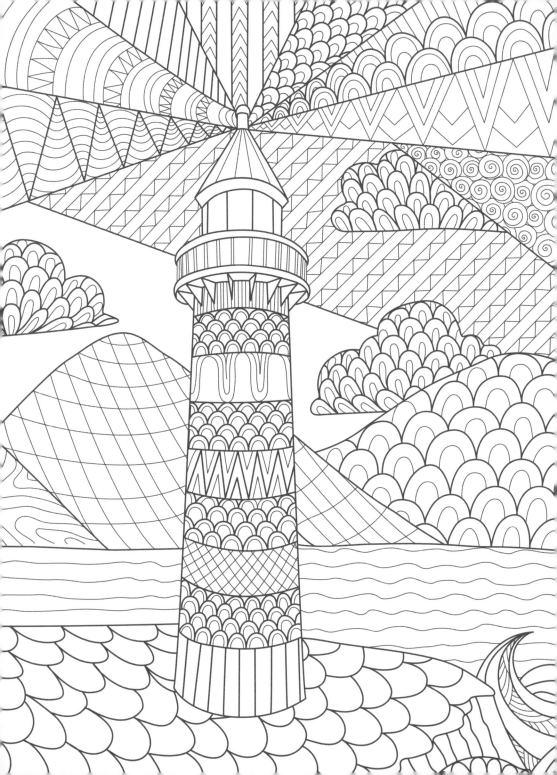

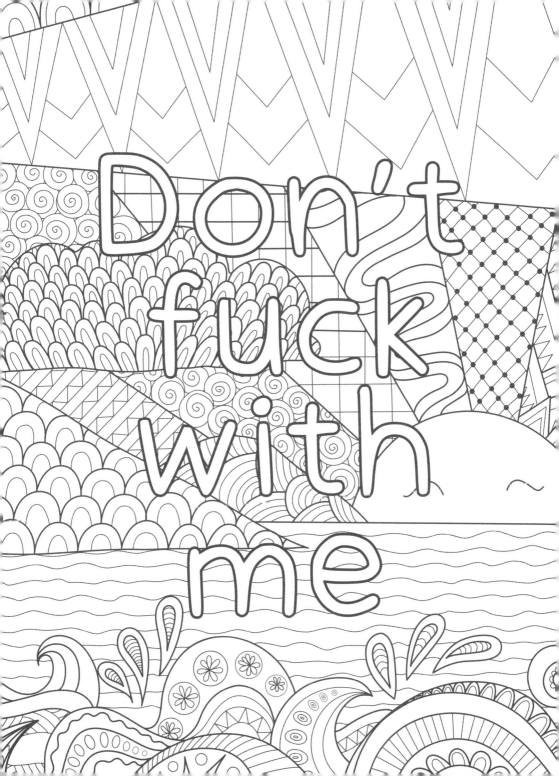

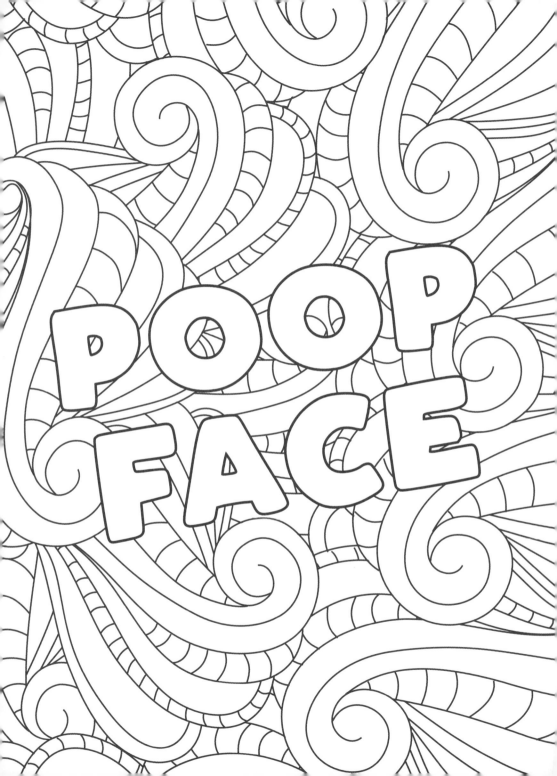

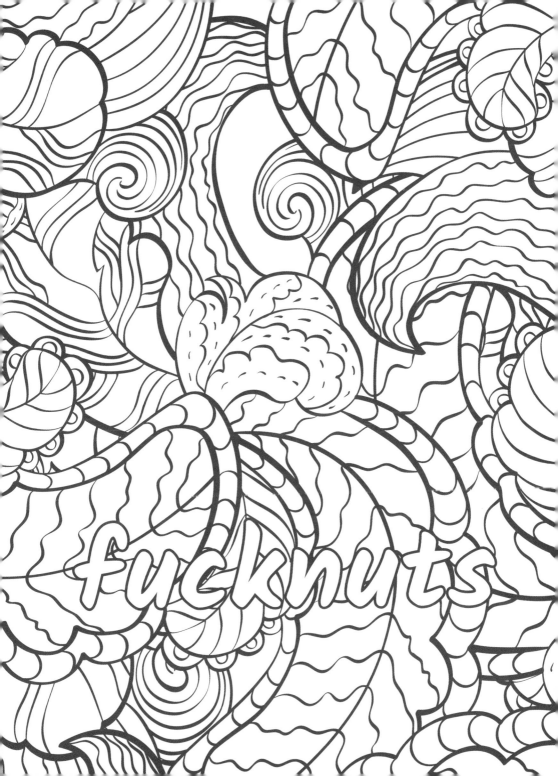

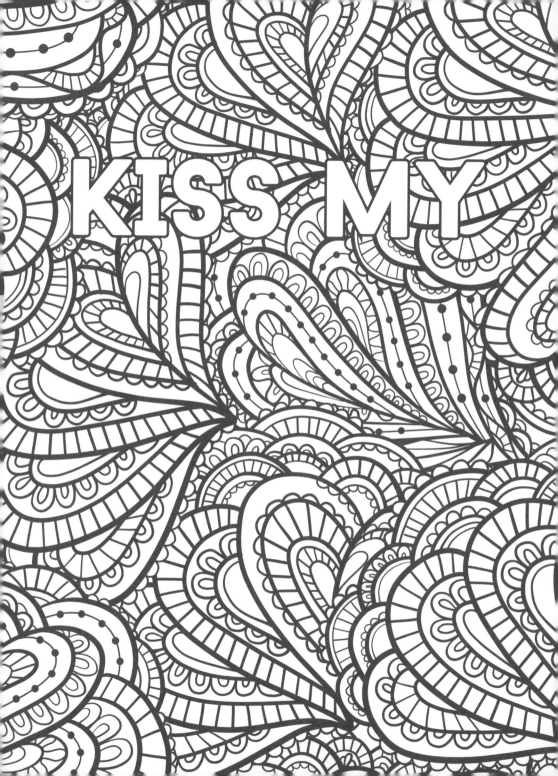

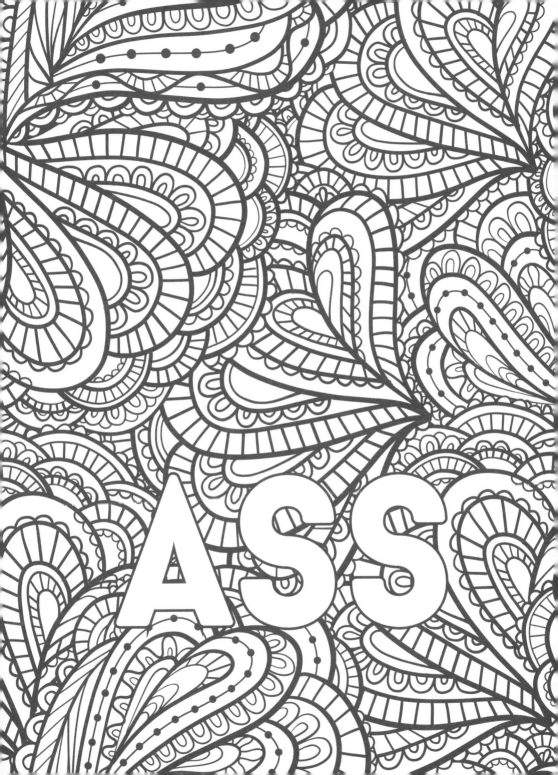

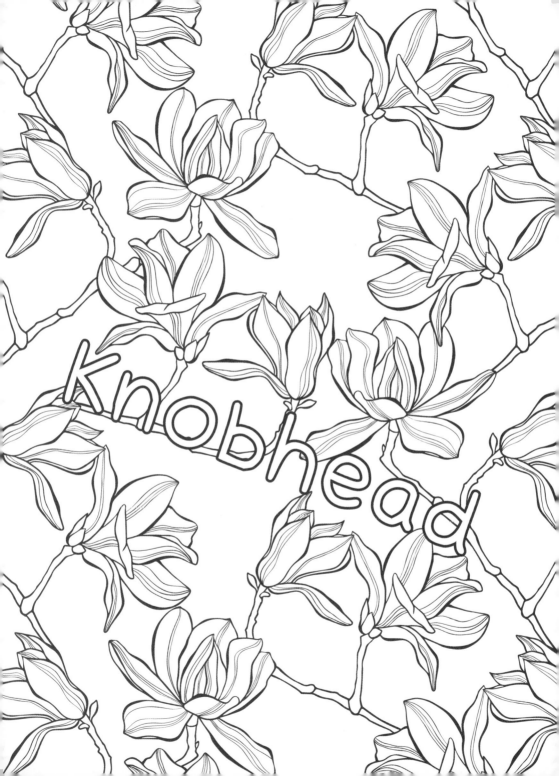

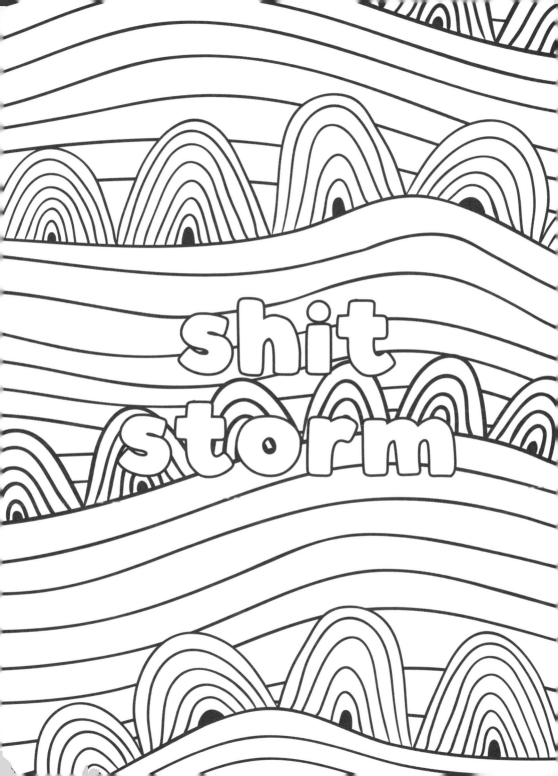

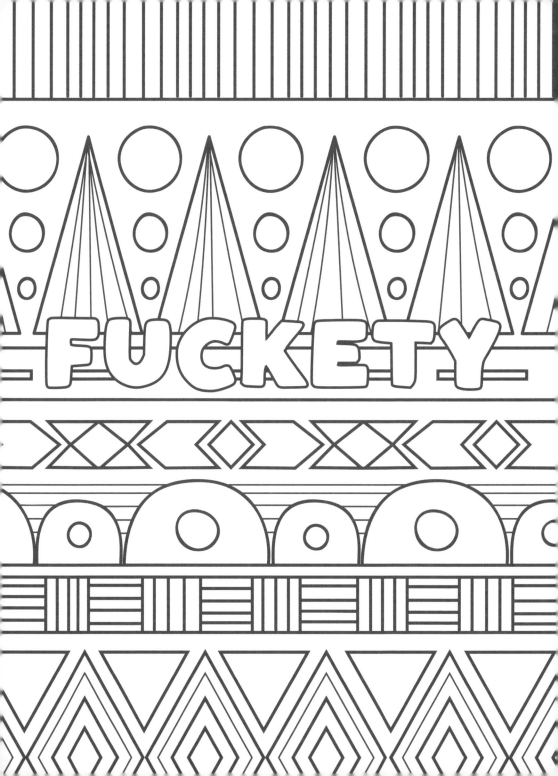

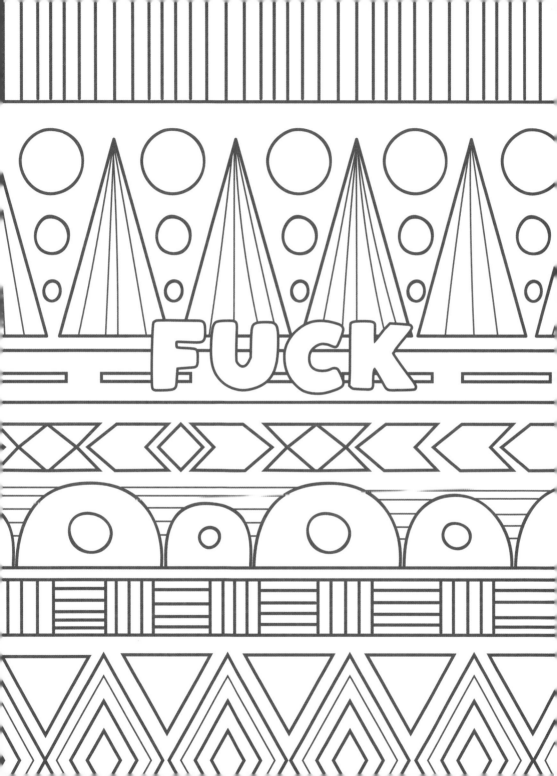

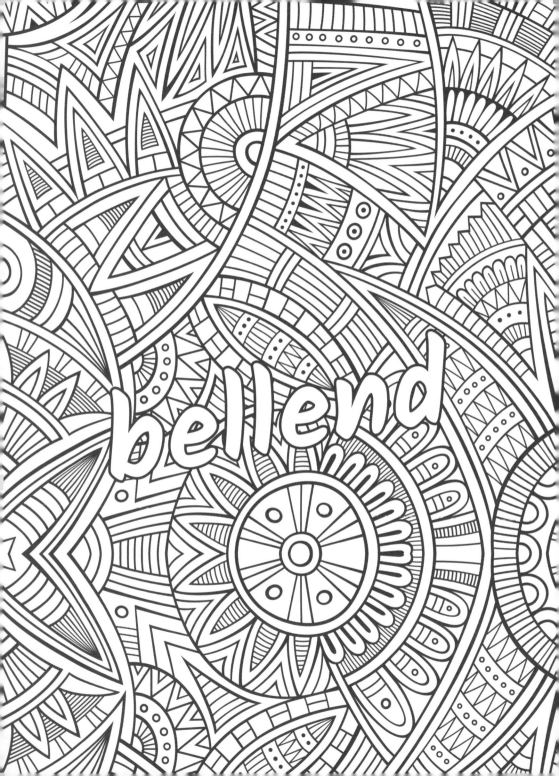

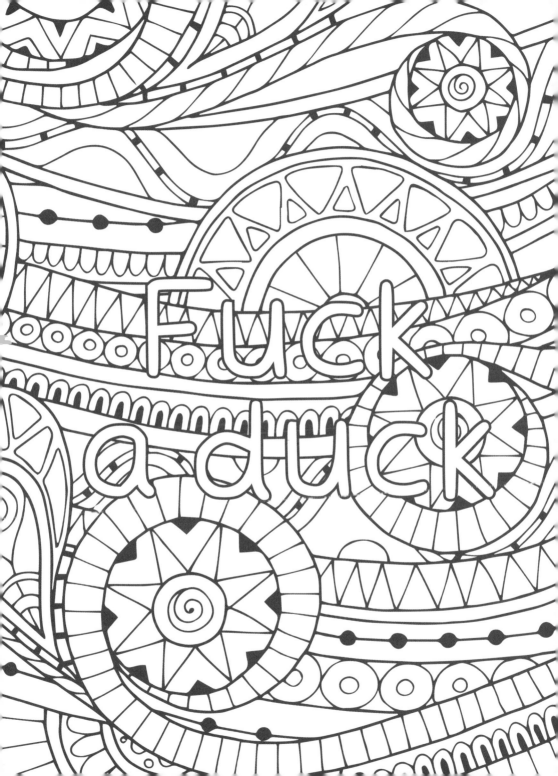

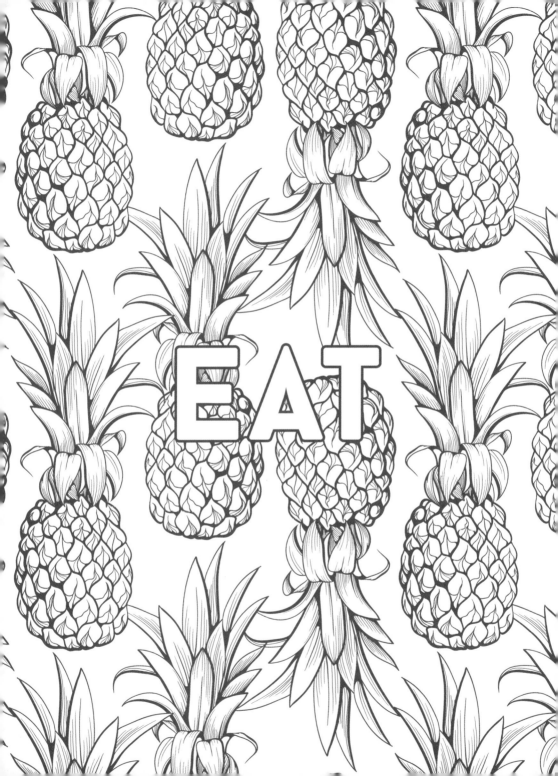

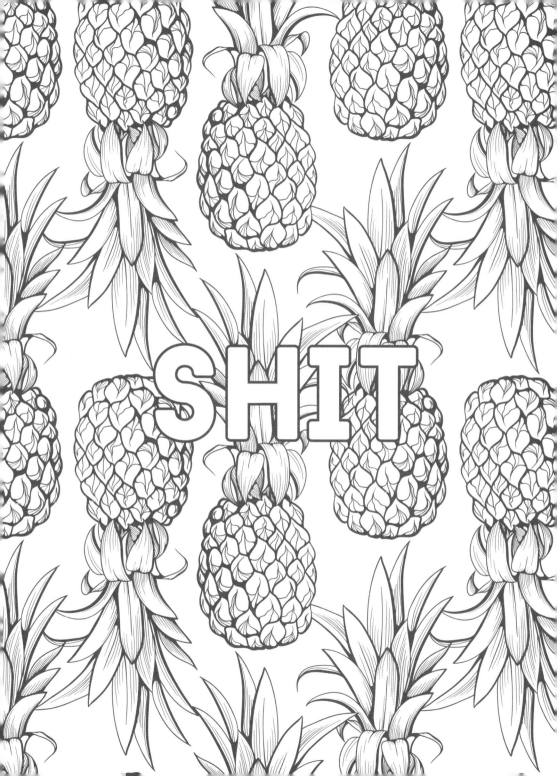

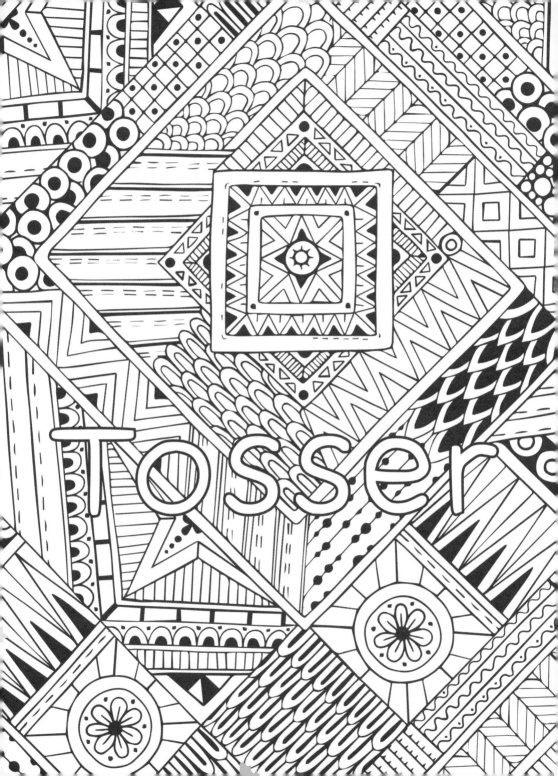

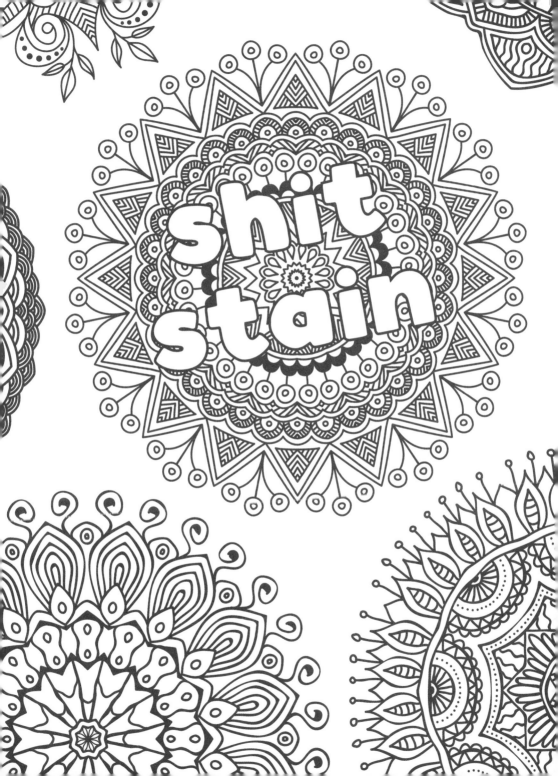

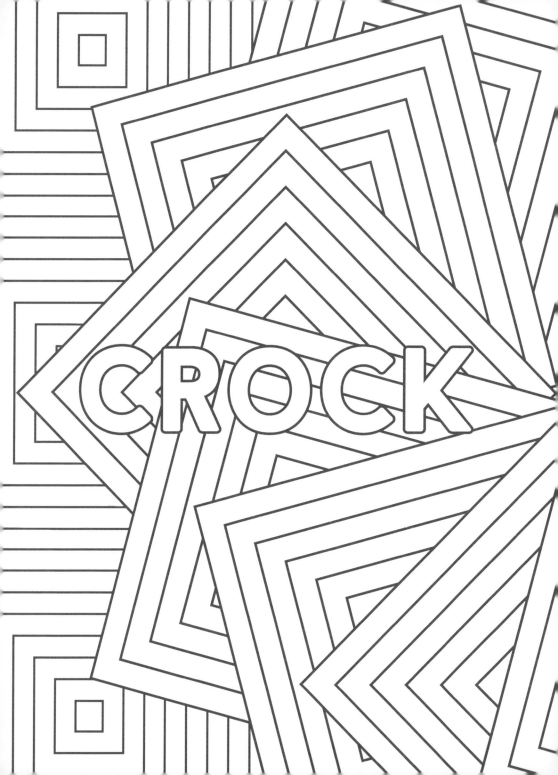

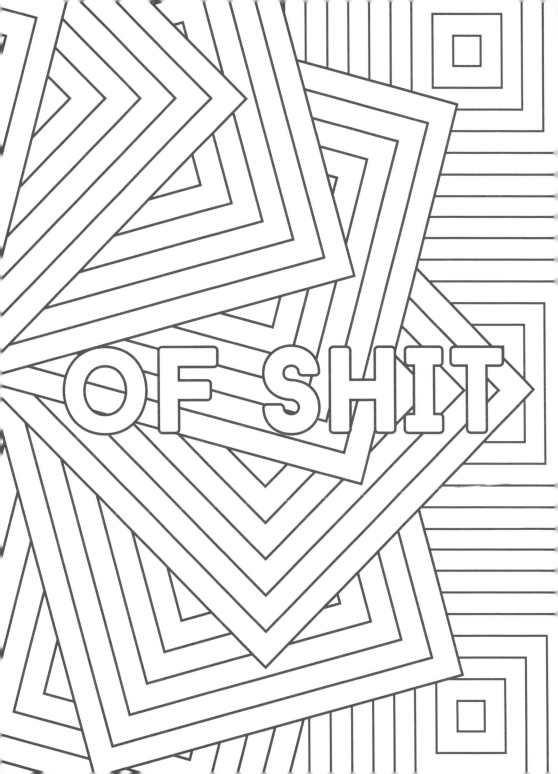

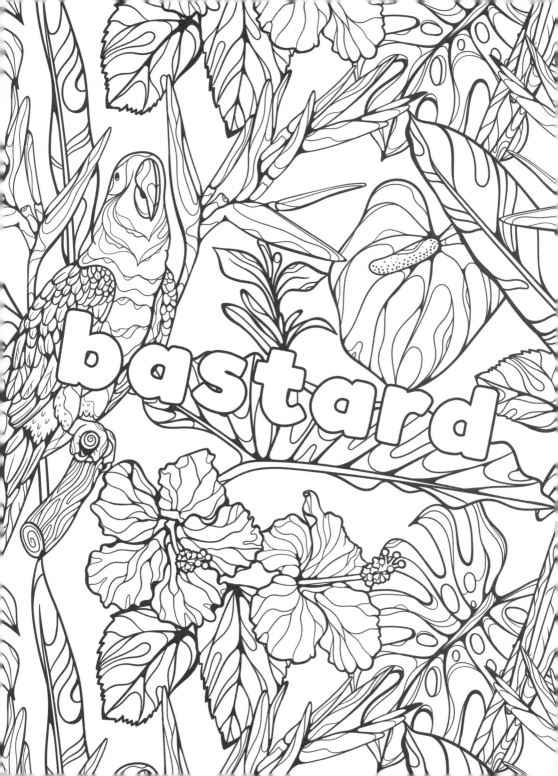

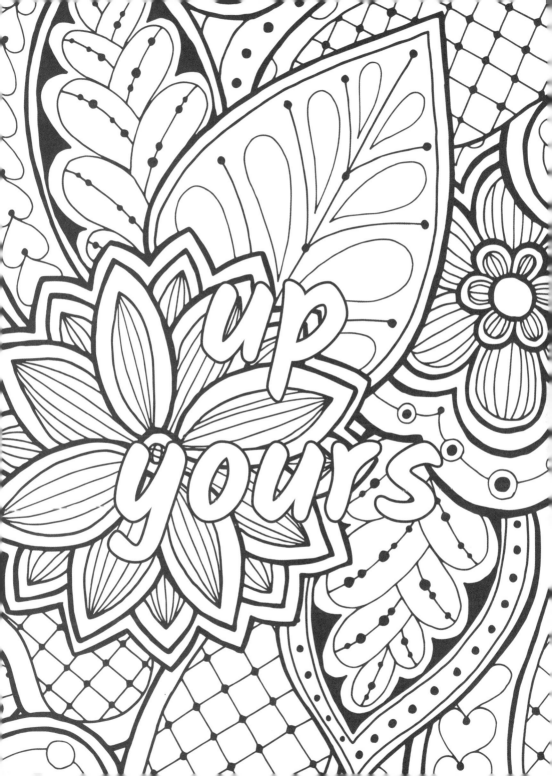

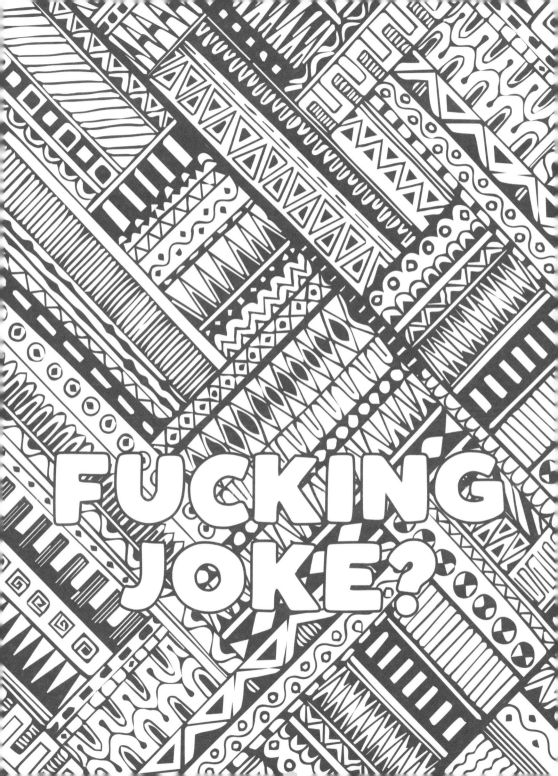

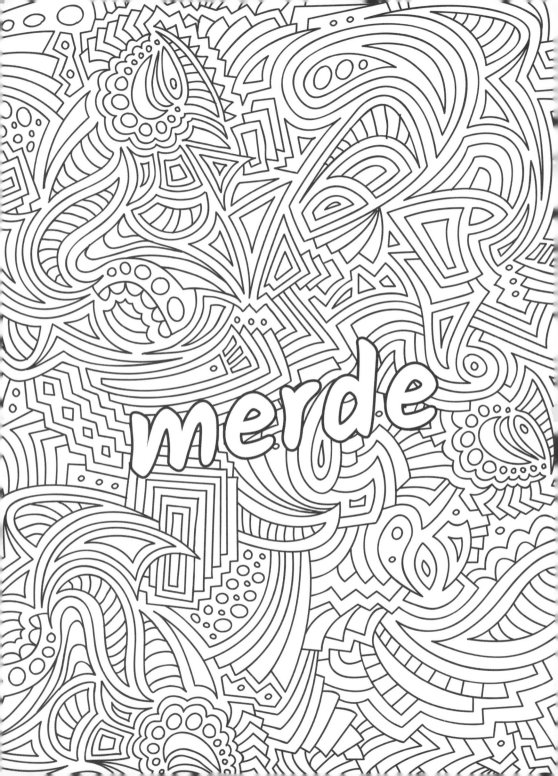

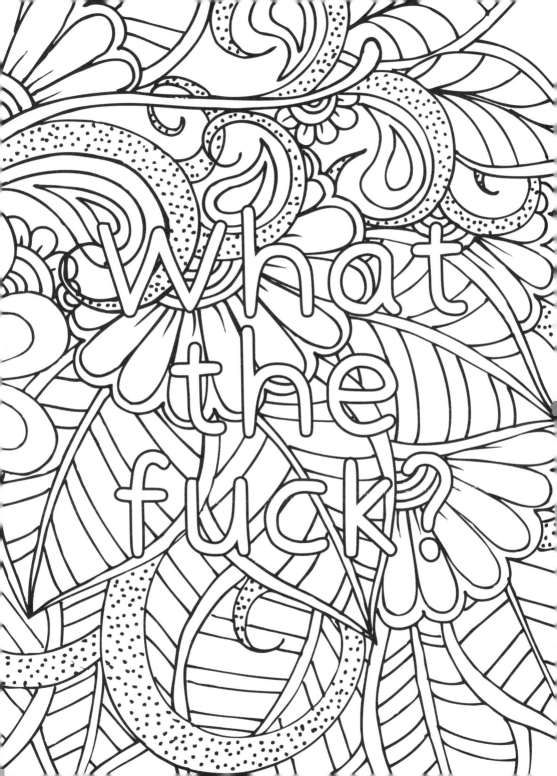

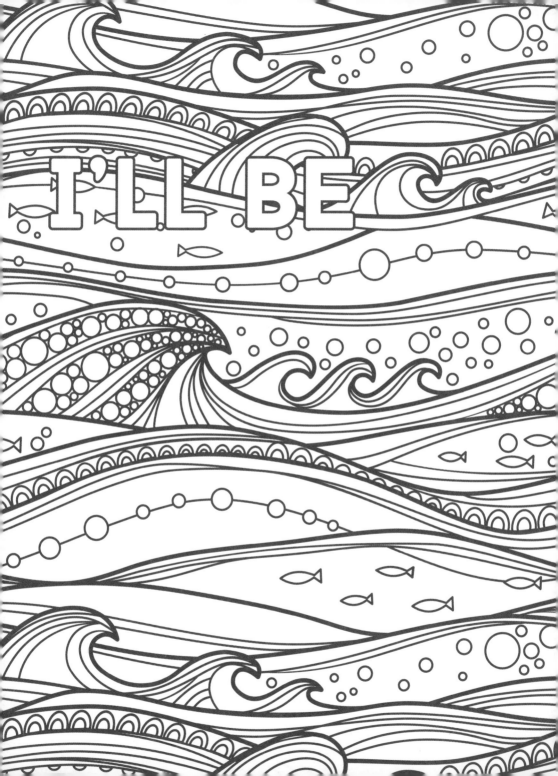

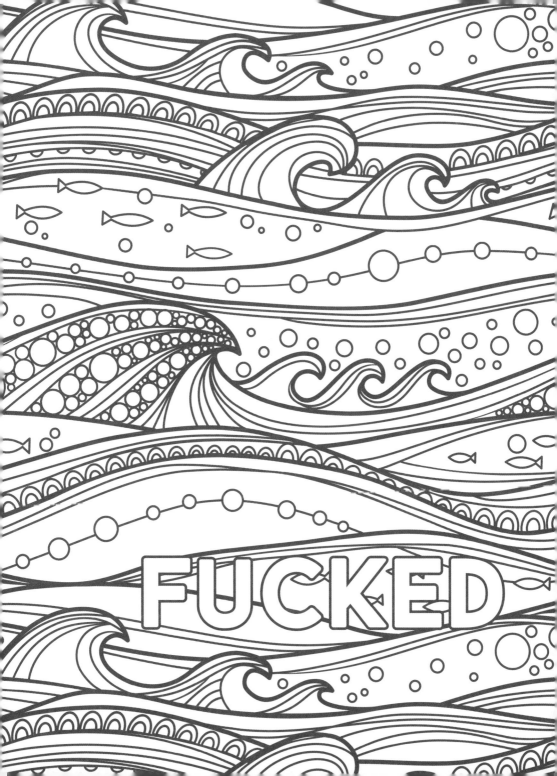

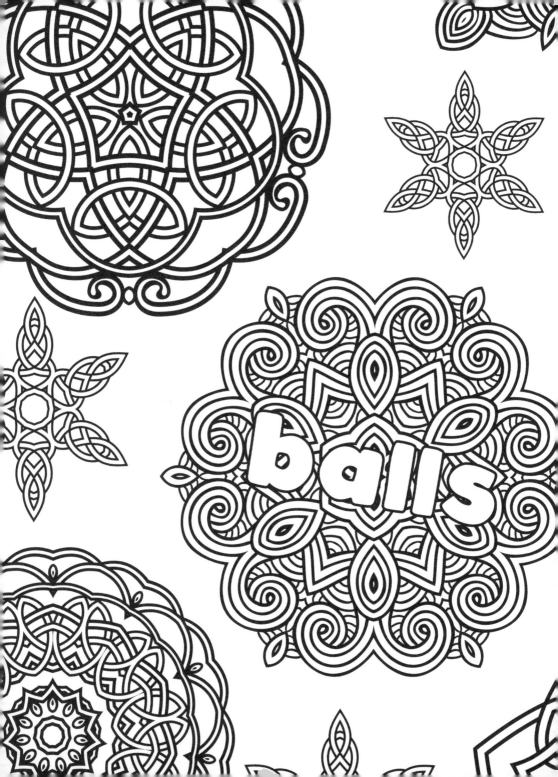

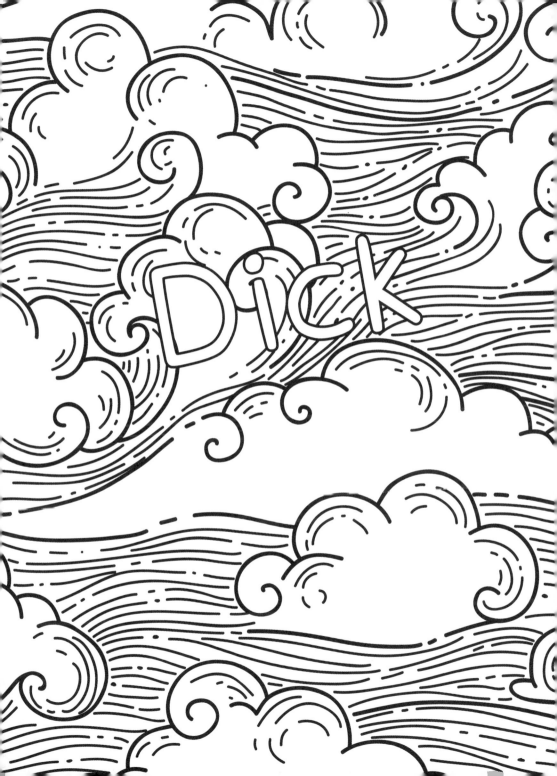

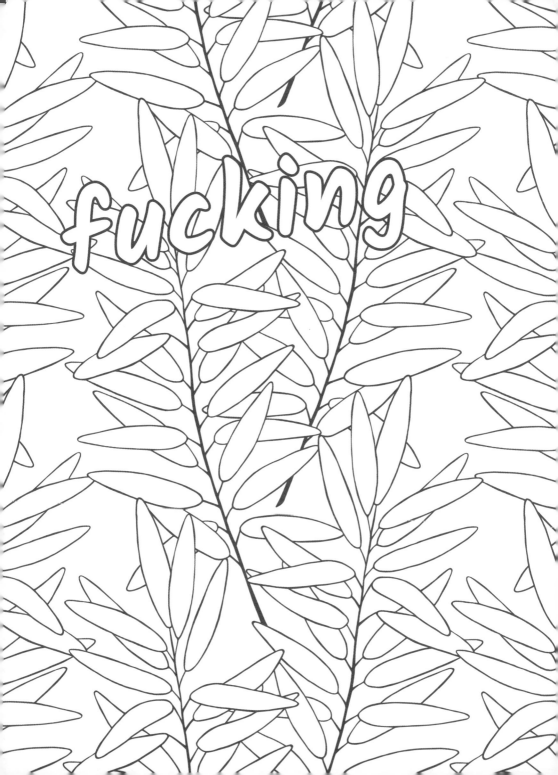

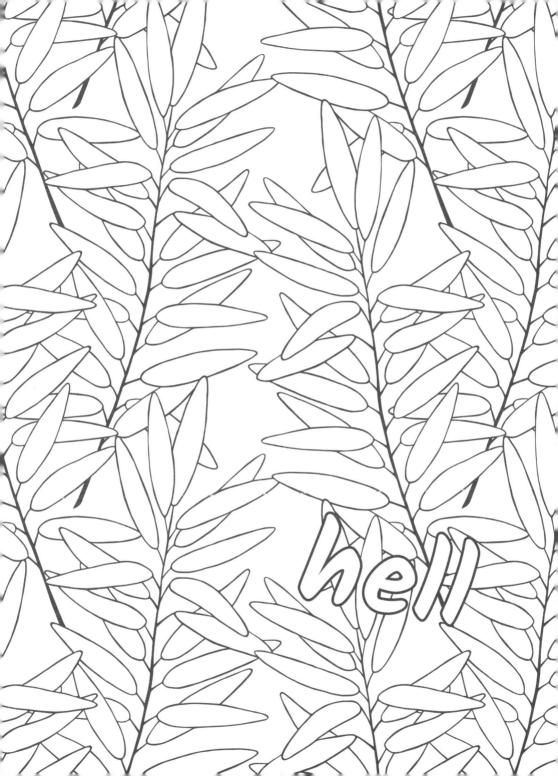

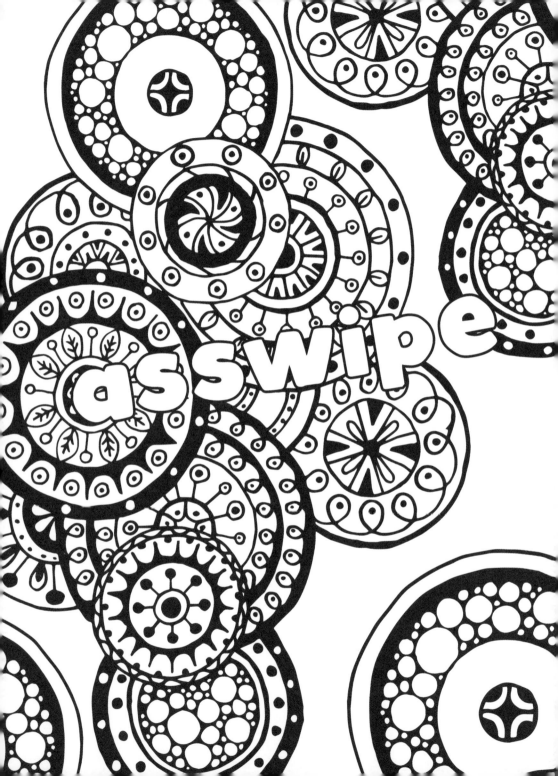

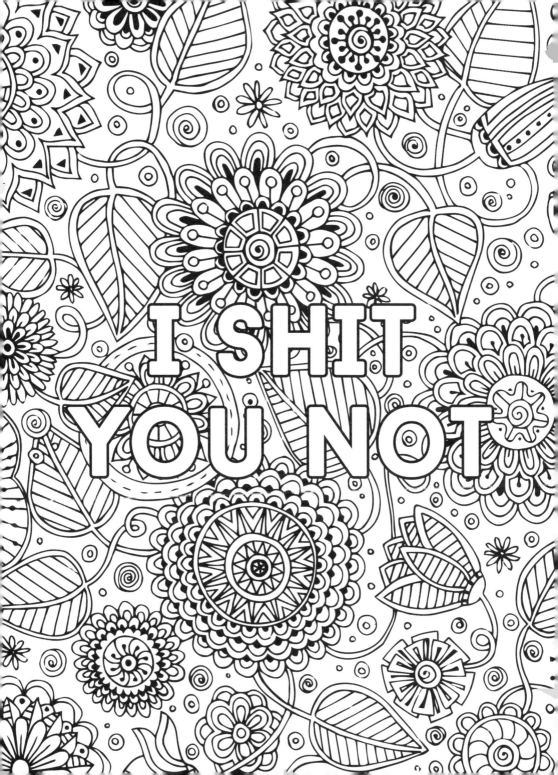

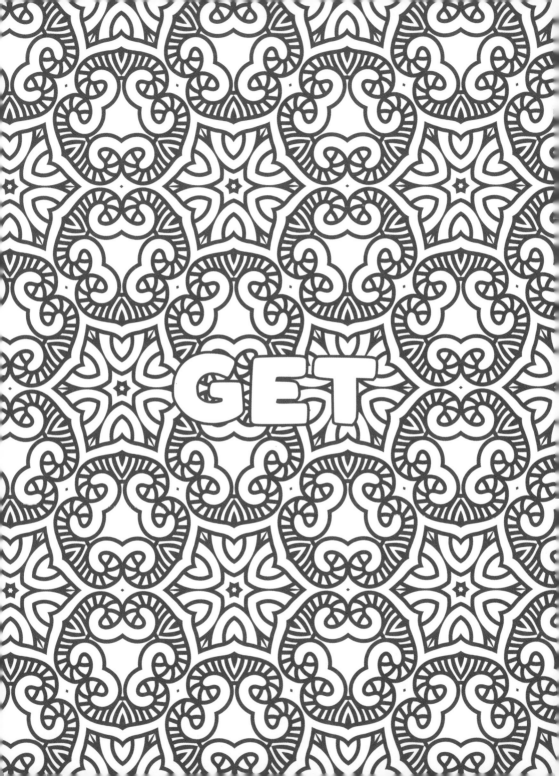

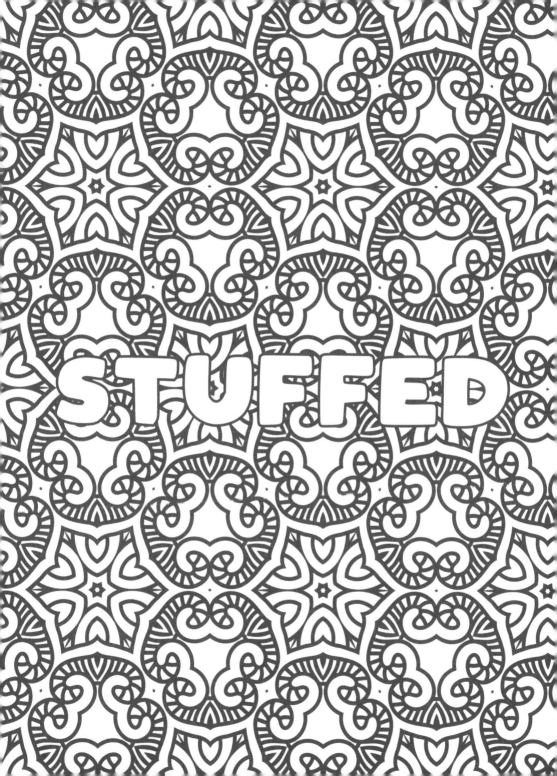

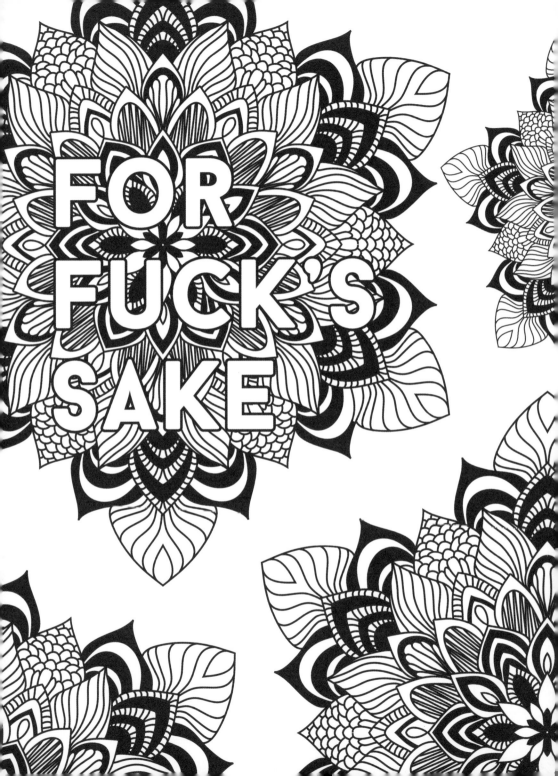

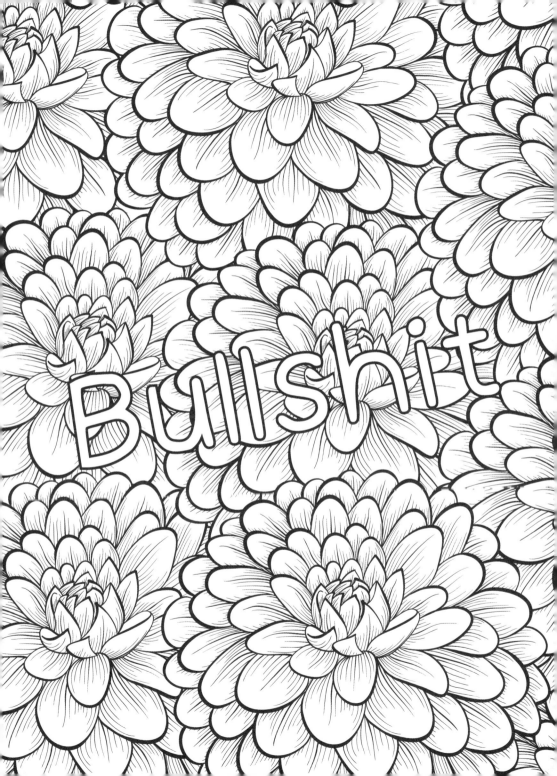

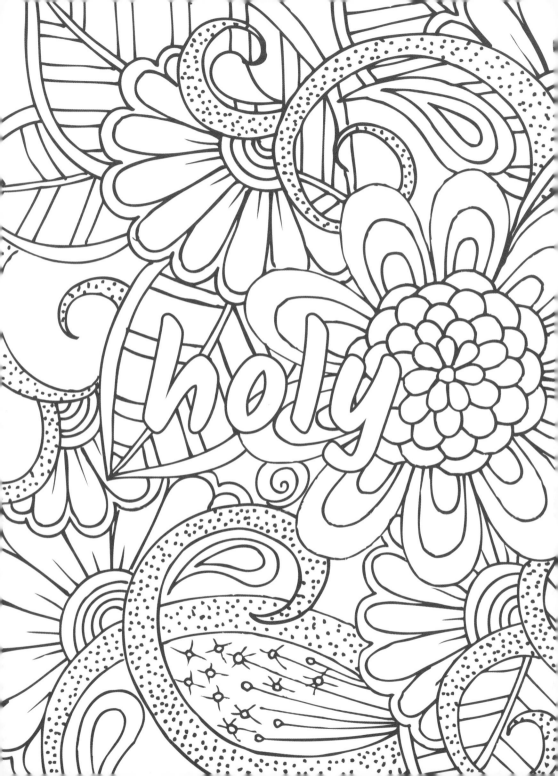

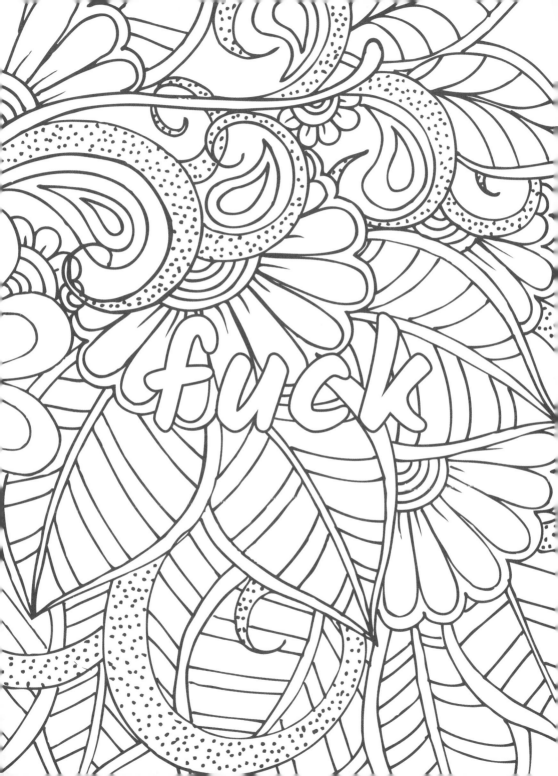

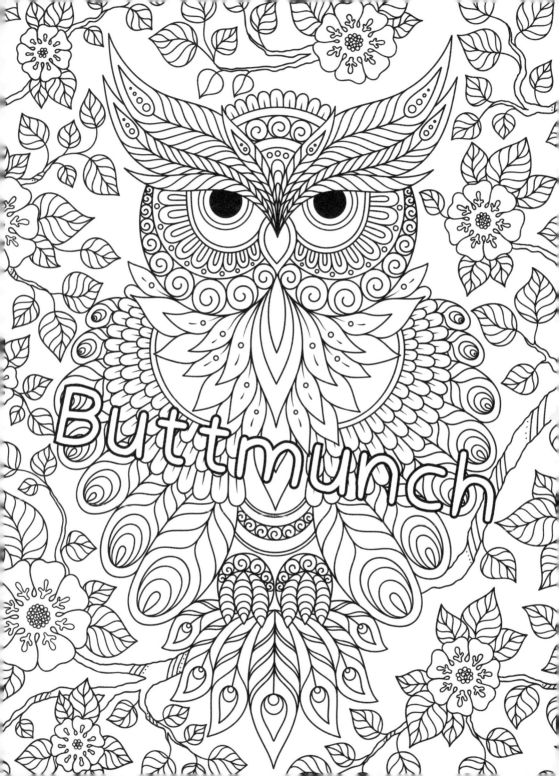

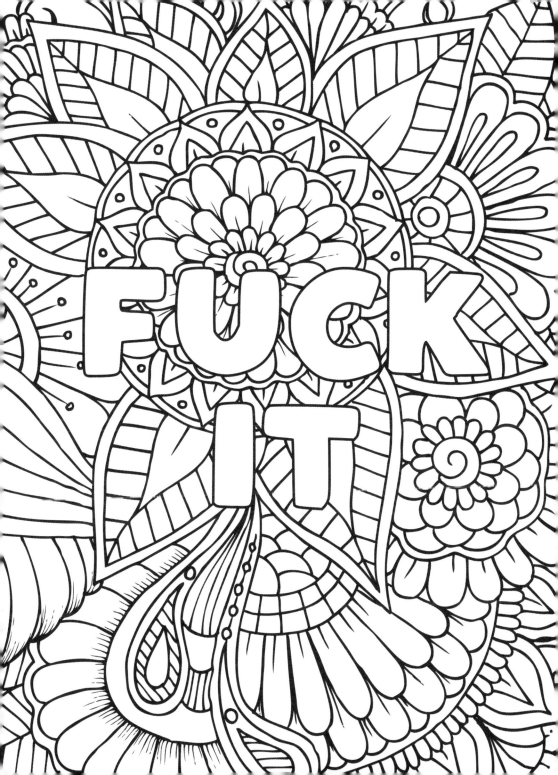

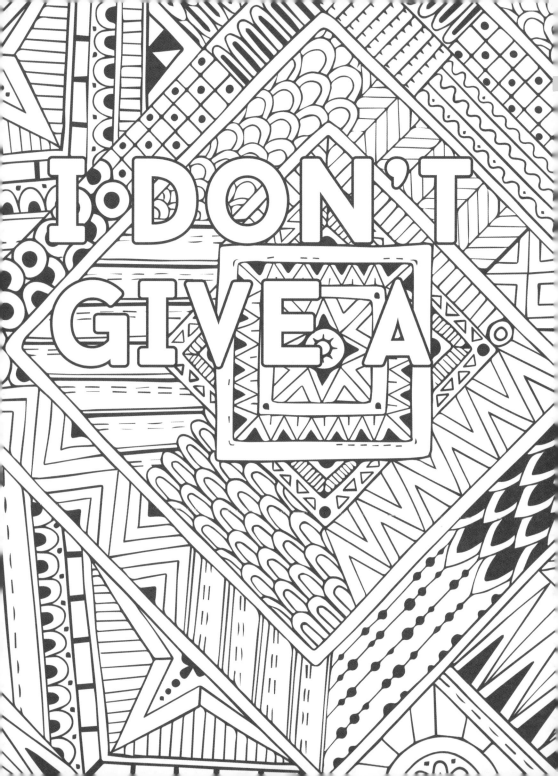

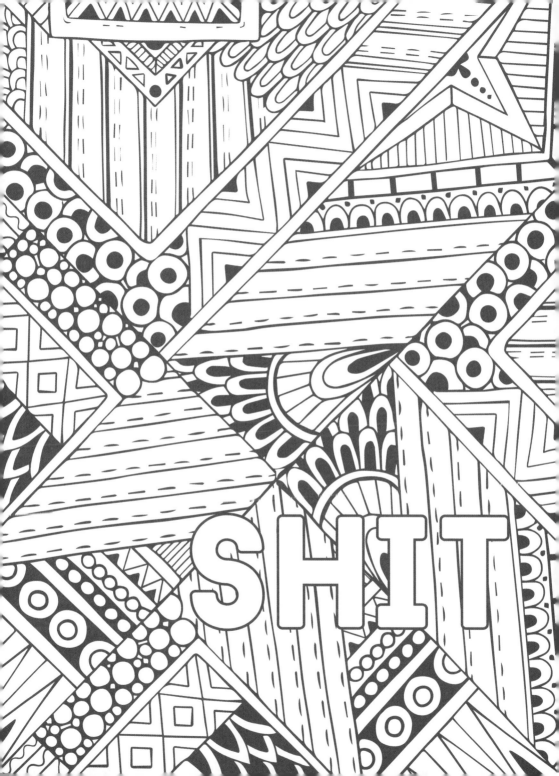

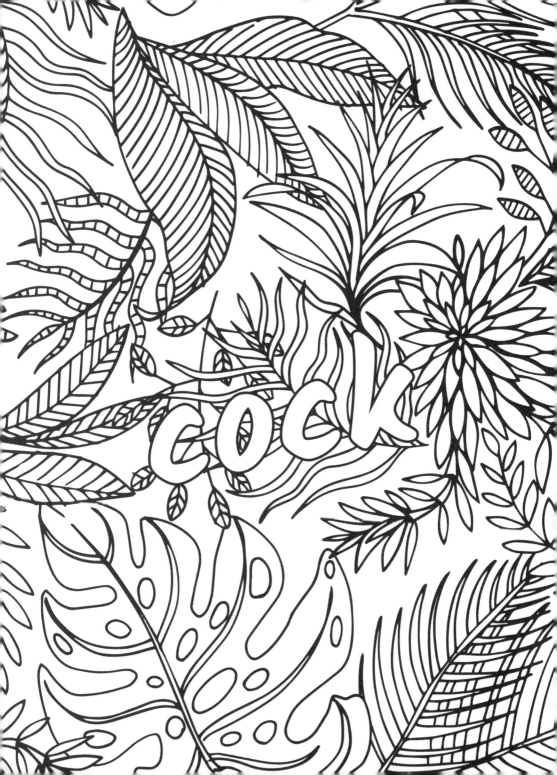

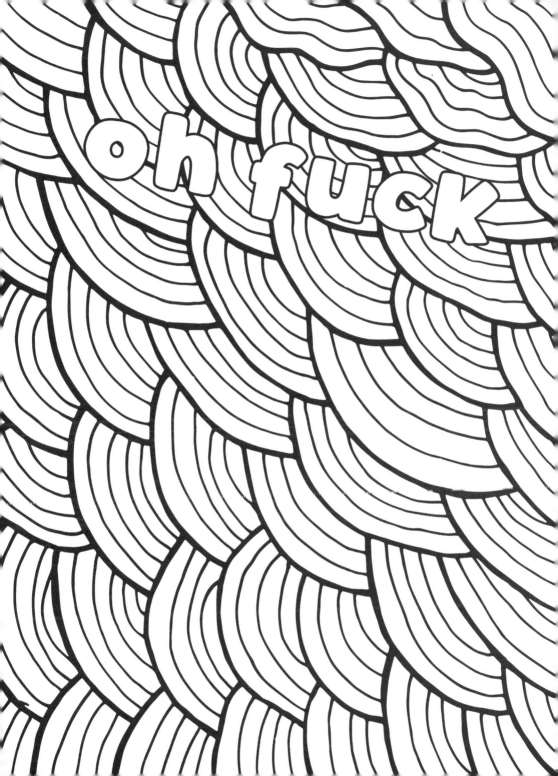

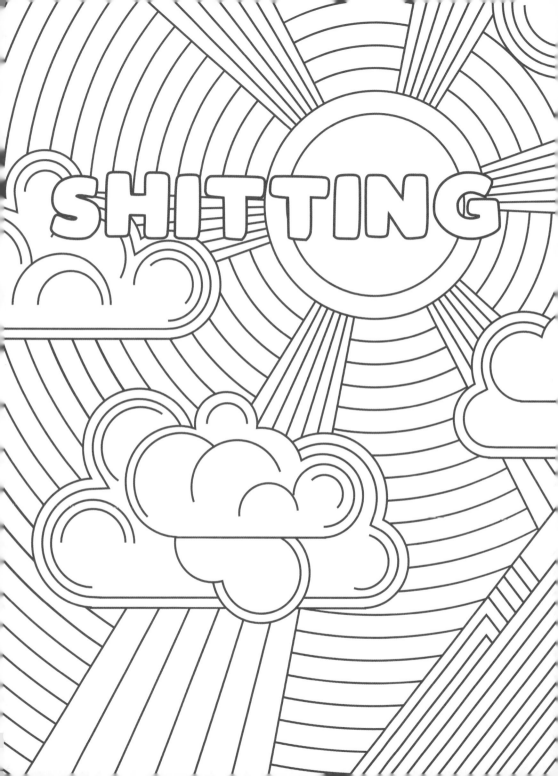

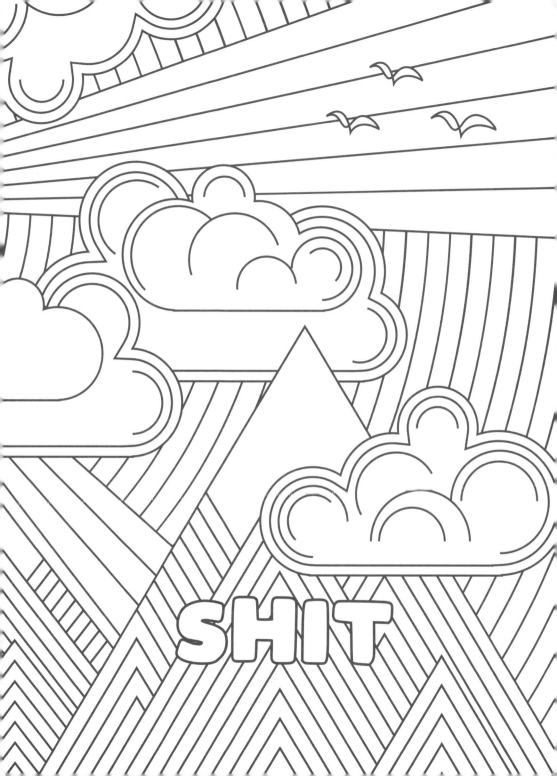

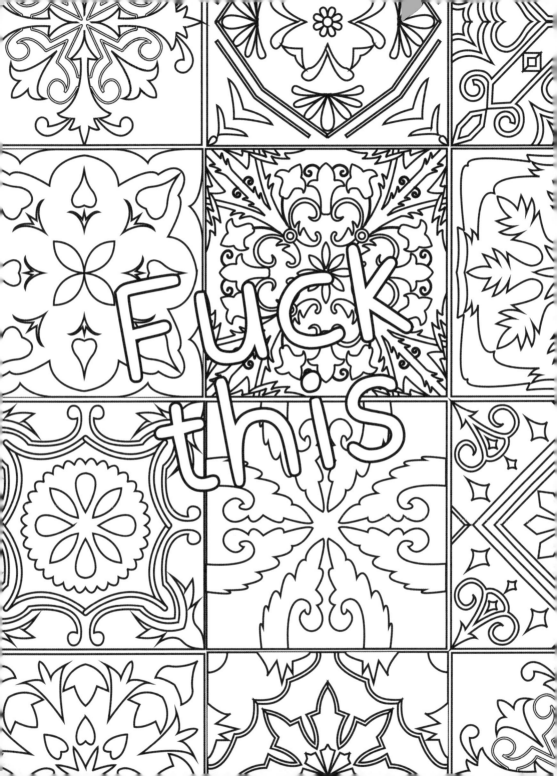

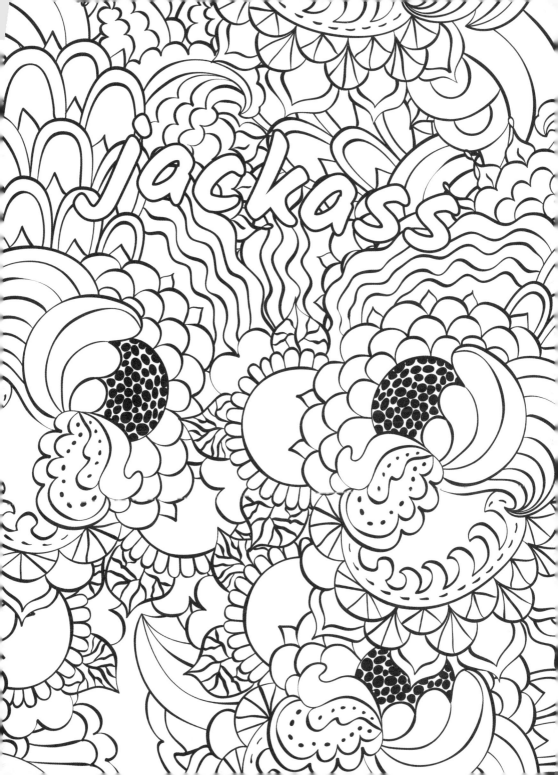

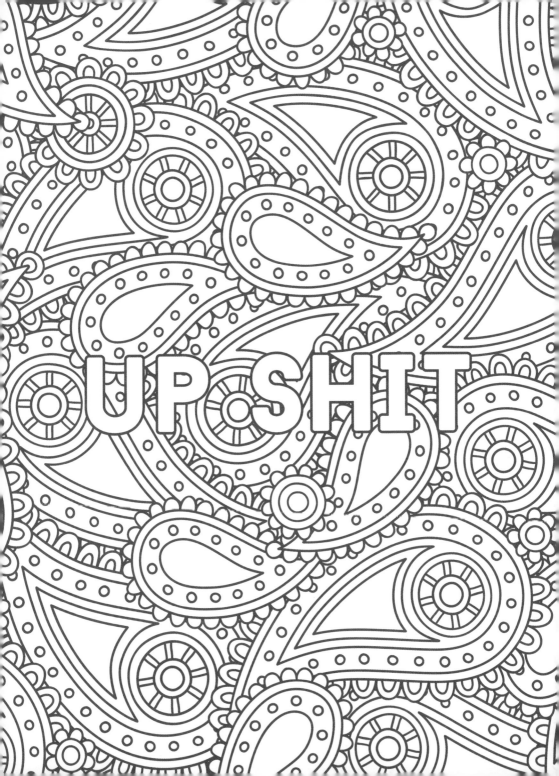

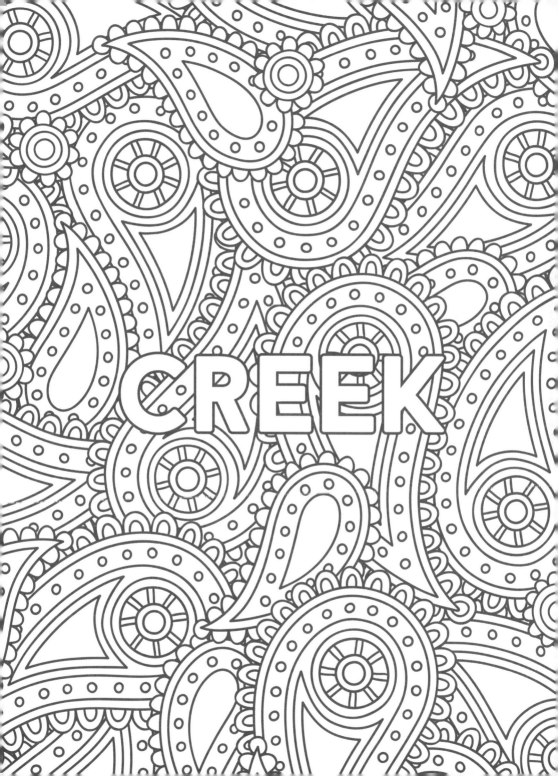

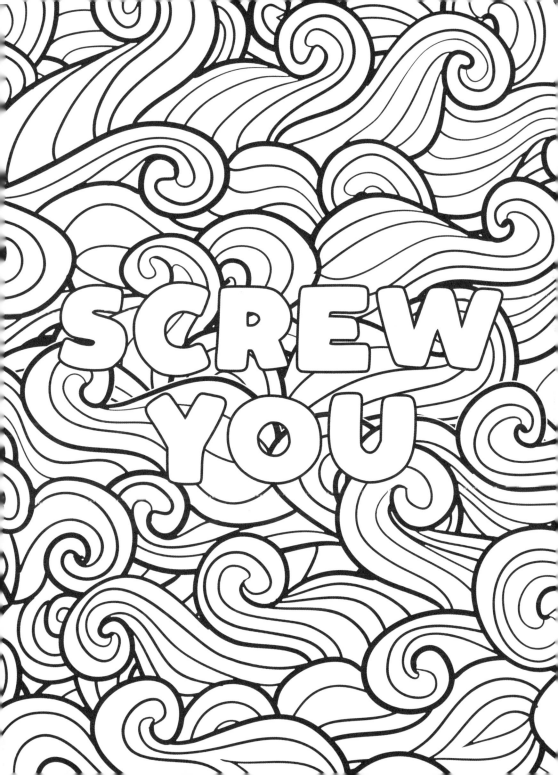

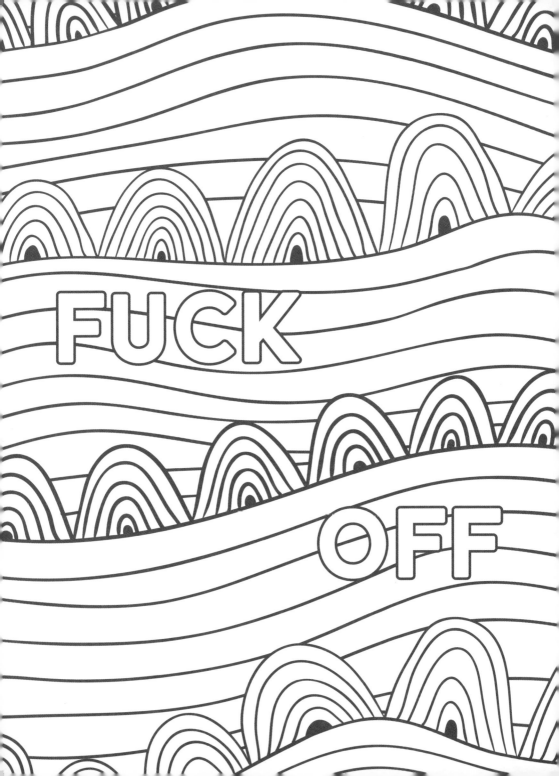

IMAGE CREDITS

If you're interested in finding out
more about our books, find us on Facebook at
Summersdale Publishers, on Twitter/X at **@Summersdale**
and on Instagram and TikTok at **@summersdalebooks**.

www.summersdale.com

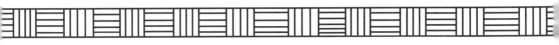

An Hachette UK Company
www.hachette.co.uk

Summersdale Publishers
Part of Octopus Publishing Group Limited
Carmelite House
50 Victoria Embankment
LONDON
EC4Y 0DZ
UK

www.summersdale.com

Printed and bound in the UK by Bell & Bain Ltd, Glasgow

ISBN: 978-1-78783-995-3

This FSC® label means
that materials used for
the product have been
responsibly sourced

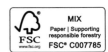

MIX
Paper | Supporting
responsible forestry
FSC® C007785

Substantial discounts on bulk quantities of Summersdale books are available to corporations, professional associations and other organizations. For details contact general enquiries: telephone: +44 (0) 1243 771107 or email: enquiries@summersdale.com.